Radiological Atlas of
Biliary and Pancreatic
Disease

Radiological Atlas of Biliary and Pancreatic Disease

HIRAM BADDELEY
MB BS DMRD FRCR
*Professor and Head of Department of Radiology, University of Queensland;
Formerly Consultant Radiologist, Bristol Royal Infirmary, and Clinical
Lecturer, University of Bristol*

DANIEL J. NOLAN
MB BCh BAO MRCP DMRD FRCR
*Consultant Radiologist, The Radcliffe Infirmary, Oxford; Clinical Lecturer,
University of Oxford*

PAUL R. SALMON
BSc(Hons) MB BS FRCP FRCPE
*Senior Lecturer in Medicine, University of Bristol; Honorary Consultant
Physician, Bristol Health District (Teaching)*

with contributions by

E. RHYS DAVIES MA MB BChir DMRD FRCR FRCPE, *Consultant
Radiologist, Bristol Royal Infirmary; Clinical Lecturer, University of
Bristol;*
F. G. M. ROSS MB BCh BAO DMRD FRCR FFR (RCSI), *Consultant
Radiologist, Bristol Royal Infirmary; Clinical Lecturer, University of
Bristol;*
GORDON EVISON MB BS DMRD FRCR, *Consultant Radiologist, Royal
United Hospitals, Bath*

Foreword by

J. H. MIDDLEMISS CMG MD FRCP FRCR FRCS
Professor of Radiology, University of Bristol

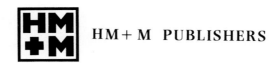

HM+M PUBLISHERS

© H. Baddeley, D.J. Nolan, P.R. Salmon 1978

First edition published by
HM+ M Publishers Ltd
Milton Road, Aylesbury
Buckinghamshire, England

0 85602 054 0

Printed in Great Britain at
the Alden Press, Oxford

Contents

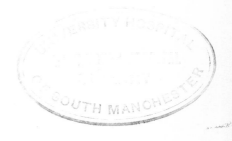

Foreword

In medicine, todays' advancing fringe when evaluated becomes tomorrow's routine practice. In radiology so much is happening, so many exciting developments are taking place, that it is sometimes too easy to forget that the majority of patients needing our expertise are those suffering from the mundane problems of trauma, chest diseases and disorders of the gastro-intestinal or biliary tracts. Most radiologists regard themselves as 'general' radiologists, perhaps with a special interest, and most carry an enormous work load. For a 'general' radiologist working in a 'general' district hospital alongside his 'generalist' physician and surgeon colleagues, it can be very difficult to pursue a special interest in depth and to keep abreast of the advancing fringes of thought, knowledge and investigational methods and interpretation. It can be equally difficult to evaluate in practical everyday clinical practice all that may be published in a field such as upper abdominal disorders affecting, as it does, so many patients and bringing, as it does, so much work to the radiologist.

It is important, therefore, that a book such as this present publication on the biliary tract, produced by two of the younger recognized established radiologists who work in close collaboration with important clinical gastro-intestinal centres, together with one of the leading clinical endoscopists of the same generation, should be made available.

Dr. Baddeley and Dr. Nolan have worked together for over a decade, and the former has worked in very close clinical collaboration with Dr. Paul Salmon for the past 5–6 years. They are to be congratulated on the uniformity of pattern in the preparation of this book, a book which does in fact evaluate not only the advancing fringes, the newer techniques, but puts into perspective those older, long-standing, well-tried procedures, to which we have all been used for so long, and which we may now sometimes accept uncritically. The book has been produced in the form of an atlas, the illustrations are of good quality and comprehensive, but the accompanying text is full enough to give a critical appraisal of the techniques and clinical requirements in this very important field of work. The bibliography is full, covering all important recent contributions, and is comprehensive and up to date.

I recommend this book to all practising radiologists and to all centres undertaking the training of future radiologists.

J.H. MIDDLEMISS
January 1978

Preface

The clinical investigation of patients using radiological means is a technical extension of bedside methods of interrogation and examination. A revolution is now taking place in gastroenterology as a consequence of improved roentgenological and endoscopic techniques which can give precise information about the nature and extent of pathology prior to surgical exploration.

Pathological calcification of the gallbladder, opaque stones or gas in the biliary system may be evident on plain abdominal radiographs but in the majority of subjects artificial contrast agents must be introduced. Oral cholecystography has been performed for many years and is the most commonly used investigation for suspected gallbladder lesions; none the less, it is still undergoing reappraisal and modification. Intravenous cholangiography has been improved by the use of slow infusion and safer contrast media. Introduction of contrast medium into the biliary system following endoscopic cannulation or percutaneous needle puncture has proved valuable in defining pathology and has allowed unnecessary laparotomy to be avoided in many patients.

Radiological visualization of the pancreas has been an elusive goal for a long time but at last endoscopic pancreatography and pancreatic angiography allow preoperative demonstration of pancreatic lesions. Barium studies can be of use in providing indirect evidence of pancreatic disease. Computed tomography has joined scintigraphy and sonography as another non-invasive method of visualizing the liver, bile ducts and pancreas, and can be expected to have a profound effect on biliary and pancreatic diagnosis in the future.

It is the purpose of this atlas to provide a collection of biliary and pancreatic lesions as revealed by radiological methods and to suggest patterns of investigation which we hope will be of use to radiologists, physicians and surgeons concerned in the detection of biliary and pancreatic disease.

H. BADDELEY

D. J. NOLAN

P. R. SALMON

January 1978

Acknowledgements

Very many people have made contributions to this atlas but we are especially indebted to Professor J.H. Middlemiss and Professor A.E. Read for the advice and encouragement they have given. We are grateful to all our clinical colleagues who have referred their patients for investigation in both Bristol and Oxford, but especially to Dr. K.W. Heaton, Dr. S.C. Truelove, Mr. W.K. Eltringham, Mr. H. Espiner, Mr. E.G. Lee, Mr. M.H. Gough and Professor D. Johnston. The chapter on investigations would have been incomplete without the assistance of Dr. E.R. Davies, Dr. F.G.M. Ross and Dr. G. Evison, but we are also grateful to Dr. I. Gordon, Dr. M. Gibson, Dr. J. Roylance and Dr. Joan Trowell for their help.

We would like to thank Mr. Edwin Turnbull who drew the diagrams for the atlas as well as organizing the nursing aspect of many of the investigations that are illustrated; Mr. M. Harrison, Miss G. Bryan, Mrs S. Phippen, Mrs. J. Wilkinson and their staff for providing superb radiography and Miss Christina Neumann for her meticulous organization of endoscopic investigations.

Our thanks are due to the colleagues who provided radiographs, figures and tables for inclusion in the atlas—Dr. Kyaw Aung, Dr. J. Beales, Prof. M.K. Bilbao, Dr. T.A.S. Buist, Dr. R.J. Burwood, Dr. J.C. Carr, Dr. P.B. Cotton, Prof. B.J. Cremin, Dr. E.R. Davies, Dr. R.D. Dick, Dr. G. Evison, Dr. E.W.L. Fletcher, Dr. P.B. Galvin, Dr. I.R.S. Gordon, Dr. P.G. Guyer, Dr. H. Herlinger, Dr. J.G. Kenny, Dr. D.J. Lintott, Mr. R.E. May, Dr. D.J. Mackenzie-Crooks, Prof. J.H. Middlemiss, Dr. J. G. McNulty (from *Radiology of the Liver*—publ. Saunders), Dr. J.F. Rey, Dr. J. Roylance, Dr. M.L. Wastie, Prof. G.H. Whitehouse and Dr. F.W. Wright. The editors of the *British Journal of Radiology*, *Clinical Radiology*, *American Journal of Roentgenology*, *Endoscopy*, *British Journal of Surgery*, *Gastroenterology*, and *X-Ray Focus* (Ilford Ltd) kindly allowed us to reproduce material from their journals, as did also the Royal College of Physicians from *11th Symposium on Advanced Medicine* (Pitman Medical).

We are especially grateful to Mrs. V. McCarthy and Mrs. R. Nolan for preparing the typed manuscript and to Mr. J. Hancock for photographic advice. Last but not least we wish to thank Mr. Patrick West of HM + M Publishers for his courtesy and co-operation.

Biliary tract disorders are difficult to consider in isolation from liver disease, with which they are often associated. Taken as a whole hepatobiliary disease encompasses a wide range of disorders, including congenital and acquired disease, inflammatory, neoplastic, traumatic, parasitic and apparently spontaneous disorders, as well as a number of uncommon diseases whose aetiology is largely unknown. Investigation of these disorders has become increasingly complex with many advances having taken place in the last few years. Radiology can fairly be said to encompass the majority of these techniques, but careful clinical examination should always precede even simple radiological investigations in order to decide which procedures are more likely to produce the diagnosis and, therefore, in which order they should be performed.

The clinical picture of biliary tract disease is represented by relatively few signs and symptoms which reflect the limited number of ways that abdominal disease can present. Thus abdominal pain or discomfort, jaundice, fever and rigors associated with abdominal pain, tenderness, and distension constitute more than three quarters of the clinical evidence. As with other diseases, however, the mode of onset of these symptoms and the association of the resulting syndrome with other clinical facets such as age, sex, family history, coexisting disease and previous surgery allows at least a differential diagnosis to be constructed, and often an accurate clinical diagnosis. In either case confirmation by radiology is normally required, since the majority of patients with biliary tract disease require surgery.

Careful clinical analysis of each symptom should be made on a knowledge of applied anatomy and disease-association. In acute cholecystitis, for example, abdominal pain may be due to gallbladder distention (deep central, visceral pain without muscle rigidity), peritoneal irritation (superficial pain with skin tenderness, hyperaesthesia and muscle rigidity both in the right hypochondrium and in the right infra-scapular region), spinal nerve pain (referred to the diaphragm, to the back and to the right hypochondrium) and digestive system pain (abdominal colic). Chronic cholecystitis, on the other hand, may be more difficult to define clinically because of ill-defined symptoms such as abdominal distention, epigastric discomfort relieved by belching, nausea (usually without vomiting) and sometimes a dull constant ache in the right hypochondrium and sub-scapular region, or even substernally or in the right shoulder.

All grades of symptoms are found in clinical practice so that it is the supporting evidence that aids the diagnosis. For example, the presence of fever, a tender gallbladder and leucocytosis would indicate acute cholecystitis; an ill toxic patient would indicate acute gangrenous cholecystitis, whilst an afebrile relatively fit patient with a positive Murphy's sign and localized tenderness in the right hypochondrium would suggest chronic cholecystitis or cholelithiasis.

In the presence of cholestatic jaundice and cholangitis (right hypochondrial pain, fever, rigors and jaundice), especially where the patient is elderly, obese, and gives a history of flatulent dyspepsia, choledocholithiasis would be more likely. Cholestatic jaundice following cholecystectomy may indicate a residual common duct calculus or a traumatic biliary stricture, whilst pain with or without mild jaundice may be due to a long cystic duct remnant, an amputation neuroma, papillary stenosis, pancreatitis or biliary dyskinesia.

1 The Clinical Presentation of Biliary Disease

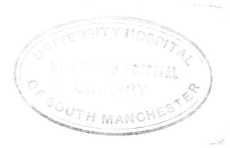

Biliary fistulae, whether post-operative or associated with gallstones, may give rise to hyponatraemia, and a metabolic acidosis (following loss of sodium and bicarbonate), gallstone ileus (nausea, abdominal colic and distention), or diarrhoea in the case of a cholecystocolic fistula (bacterial deconjugation of bile salts).

Very rarely, a hepatic duct/portal vein fistula will result in bilaemia, shock, bile pulmonary embolism and death, or a syndrome of abdominal pain, jaundice and haematemesis may be due to haemobilia. Once again it is the constellation of signs and symptoms that gives the clue, not the individual features.

Bile duct occlusion may be due either to extrinsic or to intrinsic malignant disease. Clinically, the presence of cholestatic jaundice, abdominal pain together with a variable history of weight loss, deterioration of health and anorexia, give the clue. Diarrhoea due to bile salt deficiency and haematemesis or melaena due to duodenal ulceration may also be present. In patients with carcinoma of the pancreas, completely pain-free jaundice is unusual.

The site of obstruction is of paramount importance in assessing the management and prognosis and here radiological findings are significant. Clinical support is, however valuable. For example, a patient with a history of progressive loss of weight and of cholestatic jaundice in which pruritus followed the development of jaundice, would be more likely to have an intrahepatic bile duct carcinoma than if the pruritus preceded the jaundice. In the latter case a diagnosis of primary biliary cirrhosis is more likely and a liver biopsy and mitochondrial immuno-fluorescence should be performed.

Hepatobiliary associations with other diseases are important. For example, gallstones are associated with pancreatitis, diabetes, obesity and haemolytic disease, whilst inflammatory bowel disease, usually a long-standing mild total colitis or large bowel Crohn's disease, may be associated with sclerosing cholangitis, pericholangitis or carcinoma of the bile ducts or gallbladder. Ileal Crohn's disease or ileal resection may be associated with gallstones.

Laboratory investigations and bedside procedures will often give supporting evidence and in some cases confirm the diagnosis. Anaemia may not always be due to gastrointestinal haemorrhage (e.g. in bile duct carcinoma). A leucocytosis supports a diagnosis of cholangitis and should be followed by blood cultures to exclude Gram-negative septicaemia, whilst in biliary fistulae electrolyte and acid–base balance should be determined.

Where jaundice occurs, liver function tests will determine whether the jaundice is cholestatic (raised total and conjugated bilirubin, and liver alkaline phosphatase) but alkaline phosphatase may be out of proportion to the level of serum bilirubin. In most cases and always prior to endoscopic retrograde cholangio-pancreatography a jaundiced patient should have a blood test for hepatitis B surface-antigen (HB_sA_g), and sometimes for hepatitis B surface-antibody (HB_sAB). Mitochondrial antibodies should be tested for in patients with persistent cholestatic jaundice, and are present in 98 per cent. of cases of primary biliary cirrhosis as well as in 30 per cent. of cases of chronic active hepatitis or cryptogenic cirrhosis. A needle liver biopsy is the fourth important procedure that may be performed before subjecting the patient to radiological procedures. It can be of value in the differential diagnosis of jaundice, although its use should be equated with the risk of inducing biliary peritonitis. It may check the diagnosis of cirrhosis and indicate the type (e.g. primary biliary cirrhosis) aid in the diagnosis and prognosis of liver injury following alcohol, drugs and virus hepatitis, or clinch the diagnosis of hepatic tumours, reticulo-endothelial disorders and chronic specific granulomas (e.g. tuberculosis, brucellosis). It may also be employed to assess the response to therapy (e.g. steroids) and to obtain liver tissue for liver enzyme studies (e.g. bilirubin glucuronyl transferase in Gilbert's disease).

Where pain is a feature, serum amylase should be measured and in all cases where acute pancreatitis is considered, even in the absence of pain, since 5 per cent. of cases of acute pancreatitis are free from pain. A persistently raised serum amylase may suggest the presence of a pseudocyst or macroamylasaemia. Mild hyperamylasaemia may occur with biliary as well as with pancreatic disease, and occurs in about half the patients following retrograde pancreatography.

2 Radiological Investigation

The radiological demonstration of biliary and pancreatic pathology is a study in radiographic contrast because the biliary tree and pancreas are not normally outlined on the plain abdominal radiograph. Pathological calcifications of the gallbladder, opaque calculi or gas in the ducts may provide such contrast so that a preliminary plain film should be obtained prior to contrast medium studies. Pancreatography and the various methods of cholangiography may be used to display the pancreas or biliary system directly. Barium studies, especially hypotonic duodenography, may provide indirect evidence of lesions in the pancreas. Barium meal examination is safe and easy for the patient but residual barium in the colon can be an obstacle to cholangiography, pancreatic ductography, angiography, scintigraphy and ultrasonography.

If two investigations are likely to provide similar information it is sensible to attempt the one that has the lesser risk and is less invasive. Although endoscopic ductography and abdominal angiography can provide invaluable information, they should only be deployed when simpler examinations have been unable to contribute to the diagnosis.

Oral cholecystography

Oral cholecystography has proved to be an accurate method for detecting gallstones and investigating suspected gallbladder disease.

The human gallbladder was first shown radiographically by Graham & Cole in 1924 using an intravenous injection of calcium tetrabromphenolphthalein. The calcium salt was soon replaced by the sodium salt and it was discovered that a dose of 3·5 g of sodium tetraiodophenolphthalein given orally would demonstrate the gallbladder (Graham *et al*. 1925). Sodium tetraiodophenolphthalein was used until the introduction of iodoalphionic acid (Priodox) in 1940 which produced better radiographic visualization of the gallbladder with fewer toxic reactions. Iopanoic acid (Telepaque) was introduced in 1952 (Hoppe & Archer 1953) and is now widely used. Other oral contrast media in current use are sodium ipodate (Biloptin; Oragrafin Sodium), calcium ipodate (Solu-Biloptin; Oragrafin Calcium), sodium tyropanoate (Bilopaque) and iocetamic acid (Cholebrin).

Like the urographic media these biliary contrast agents are basically substituted triiodobenzoic acid compounds (Lasser 1966). Contrast media primarily excreted by the liver tend to have higher molecular weights, and do not contain a side chain at the number five position on the benzene ring. They bind strongly to serum albumen at physiological pH while the urine-directed media have completely substituted rings and have little or no conductive binding to albumen or other serum protein.

The oral contrast media are lipid soluble and are absorbed by diffusion across the intestinal mucosa. They are carried in the blood, bound to serum albumen and are transferred through the liver to the bile by an active transport process. A portion of the contrast material flows directly into the duodenum but the majority of it reaches the gallbladder, where it becomes concentrated due to reabsorption of water by the gallbladder mucosa (Berk *et al*. 1974). When the gallbladder contracts the contrast medium passes to the duodenum via the common bile duct and it is excreted in the stool with only a small amount being reabsorbed from the intestine. About 65 per cent. of iopanoic acid is excreted in the faeces and the remainder in the urine.

Unpleasant side-effects such as nausea, diarrhoea, abdominal pain and dysuria are not uncommon with oral cholecystographic agents, although skin reactions and vomiting occur infrequently (White & Fischer 1962). About 50 cases of oral cholecystographic media causing acute renal failure have been reported (Mudge 1971), a large number of which had been given bunamiodyl (Orabilex) which has now been withdrawn from use. In some of the cases where media in current use have caused renal failure, large doses of iopanoic acid were involved (Canales et al. 1969). Renal failure is more likely to occur if there is hepatobiliary disease of increasing severity, if the patient is dehydrated, or if there has been a recent intravenous cholangiogram.

A plain film of the gallbladder area should be taken some time before oral cholecystography is to be performed. The patient should take a dose of three grammes of cholecystographic medium with a light evening meal and no further solid food until after the examination on the following day. Fluids that contain neither fat nor milk should be encouraged, as they reduce even further the remote chance of renal failure and it has been shown that water can be taken in quite large quantities without any reduction in the quality of gallbladder opacification (Bainton et al. 1973). Optimum visualization of the gallbladder occurs 14–19 hours after ingestion of iopanoic acid (Whalen et al. 1972). Good radiographic technique with careful centring and collimation is essential, and a low kilovoltage of about 60–80 Kv gives the best results. Supine oblique and prone oblique views of the gallbladder should be taken, followed by erect views, best obtained by screening the patient in different positions and using compression to obtain views of the gallbladder free from overlying gas shadows. The examination is completed when a final film is taken half an hour after a fatty meal. The after-fat film is essential for the diagnosis of adenomyomatosis and cholesterolosis and is sometimes helpful in demonstrating small stones (Harvey et al. 1976).

When a poorly opacified gallbladder is obscured by overlying gas shadows, tomography may be necessary to obtain adequate views. If the gallbladder does not opacify, the film should be carefully examined for evidence of bile or intrahepatic duct opacification and tomography should be used, if necessary, to show the ducts. Bile duct opacification with non-filling of the gallbladder indicates the presence of gallbladder disease (McNulty 1975).

The gallbladder may fail to opacify for a number of reasons: the contrast medium may be trapped in pharyngeal or oesophageal diverticula; obstructive lesions such as achalasia of the cardia, carcinoma of the oesophagus or pyloric stenosis may prevent the medium from reaching the small bowel, or it may be vomited. Small-bowel diseases, malabsorption and diarrhoea are often cited as reasons for non-opacification of the gallbladder (Wise 1966; Berk 1973)

though it has been shown that patients with these conditions do absorb sufficient contrast medium to produce good opacification (Low-Beer et al. 1972). When liver function is abnormal and the serum bilirubin level is greater than 30 m mol/l the gallbladder will not opacify (Kreel 1973). The double dose examination seldom yields further information where the single dose has failed (Wise 1966; Achkar et al. 1969) and it is more likely to cause renal insufficiency (Grainger 1972; Berk 1973). However, a double dose may improve opacification when the gallbladder is only faintly outlined with a single dose.

References

Achkar E., Norton R. A. & Siber F. J. (1969) Amer. J. dig. Dis., **14**, 80

Bainton D., Davies G. T., Evans K. T., Gravelle I. H. & Abernethy M. (1973) Clin. Radiol., **24**, 381

Berk R. N. (1973) Surg. Clin. N. Amer., **53**, 973

Berk R. N., Loeb P. M., Goldberger L. E. & Sokoloff J. (1974) New Engl. J. Med., **290**, 204

Canales C. O., Smith G. H., Robinson J. C., Remmers A. R. Jnr. & Sarles H. E. (1969) New Engl. J. Med., **281**, 89

Graham E. A. & Cole W. H. (1924) J. Amer. med. Ass., **82**, 613

Graham E. A., Cole W. H. & Copher G. H. (1925) J. Amer. med. Ass., **84**, 1175

Grainger R. G. (1972) Brit. med. Bull., **28**, 191

Harvey I. C., Thwe M. & Low-Beer T. S. (1976) Clin. Radiol., **27**, 117

Hoppe J. O. & Archer S. (1953) Amer. J. Roentgenol., **69**, 630

Kreel L. (1973) Clin. Gastroent., **2**, 185

Lasser E. C. (1966) Radiol. Clin. N. Amer., **4**, 511

Low-Beer T. S., Heaton K. W. & Roylance J. (1972) Brit. J. Radiol., **45**, 427

McNulty J. G. (1975) Brit. med. J., **i**, 38

Mudge G. H. (1971) New Engl. J. Med., **284**, 929

Whalen J. P., Rizzuti R. J. & Evans J. A. (1972) Radiology, **105**, 523

White W. W. & Fischer H. W. (1962) Amer. J. Roentgenol., **87**, 745

Wise R. E. (1966) Radiol. Clin. N. Amer., **4**, 521

Intravenous cholangiography

Intravenous cholangiography is the method of choice for the radiographic demonstration of the biliary tree when the prime interest is in the examination of the bile ducts. Gallbladder opacification is also achieved in patients who have had neither cholecystectomy nor cystic duct occlusion, but it must be stressed that intravenous cholangiography should not be employed as a substitute for oral cholecystography when examination of the gallbladder only is required, because the oral method usually produces much better gallbladder opacification and is easier to perform.

The contrast media used are iodipamide methylglucamine (Biligrafin; Biligrafin Forte; Cholografin), ioglycamide methylglucamine (Biligram) and meglumine iodoxomate (Cholovue), a new contrast medium, which has recently become available (Sargent *et al.* 1975).

The iodipamide molecule contains two iodinated benzene rings linked by adipic acid, and the ioglycamide molecule differs from it in that the iodinated benzene rings are linked by diglycolic acid instead of adipic acid. Iodipamide and ioglycamide are freely soluble in aqueous solution thus enabling them to be used for intra-vascular injection. They are particularly suitable because they bind to serum proteins and contrast material with a propensity for binding to proteins is preferentially excreted in the bile (Lasser *et al.* 1962). An active transport process transfers iodipamide and ioglycamide against the gradient of a low serum level through the liver to a much higher level in the bile (Fischer 1965; Rosati & Schiantarelli 1970).

Indications Intravenous cholangiography is indicated
1 in patients who have had a previous cholecystectomy presenting with symptoms suggestive of biliary tract disease;
2 when the gallbladder or bile ducts are not outlined at oral cholecystography;
3 in the diagnosis of acute cholecystitis;
4 for the investigation of episodes of biliary colic or jaundice;
5 for the assessment of the degree of obstruction and the calibre of the bile ducts in patients with chronic pancreatitis;
6 in the investigation of suspected choledochal cysts (Han *et al.* 1969; Jones & Olbourne 1973);
7 when the presence of foreign bodies in the bile ducts is suspected (Martinez *et al.* 1971); and
8 for the assessment of the bile ducts prior to biliary tract surgery (Wise 1966).

Contraindications Combined severe liver and renal disease (Wise 1967) and monoclonal IgM paraproteinaemia (Waldenstrom's macroglobulinaemia) must be regarded as absolute contraindications for the use of intravenous biliary contrast media (Bauer *et al.* 1974).

Relative contraindications include a history of allergy to contrast media or drugs, asthma, and patients in whom hypotension would be dangerous such as those with ischaemic heart disease, and if possible, the examination should not be carried out during pregnancy. Caution is advocated in patients with cholestatic liver disease (Spent *et al.* 1969). In each case the potential benefit must be carefully weighed against the risk involved.

Technique Intravenous cholangiography should not be carried out within 48 hours of oral cholecystography because in a large number of patients the biliary tract fails to opacify and severe reactions are common if iodipamide is given before this period has elapsed (Finby & Blasberg 1964). Normal or nearly normal liver function is essential for a satisfactory examination, and the serum bilirubin level should be less than 45 m mol/l and be returning to normal levels rather than rising.

An aperient should be given on the two nights before the examination to ensure that detail of the biliary tract is not obscured by faecal and gas shadows. The patient should be well hydrated and have a light fat-free breakfast on the morning of the examination (Wise 1967; Martinez *et al.* 1971; Kreel 1973).

Emergency drugs and equipment should always be available in the room where the examination is being carried out. The contrast medium may be given as an injection over five or ten minutes, or as a slow infusion. Iodipamide as Biligrafin Forte is prepared in 20-ml ampoules containing 10 g of active agent for intravenous injection. The newer contrast agent ioglycamide (Biligram) is prepared in 30-ml ampoules containing 10·5 g for intravenous injection and 100-ml bottles containing 17 g suitable for infusion.

By using a slow infusion technique patients experience fewer unpleasant side-effects (Darnborough & Geffen 1966; Foy 1968; McNulty 1968; Nolan & Gibson 1970) and the concentration of iodipamide in the bile is increased (Whitney & Bell 1972). Recent work indicates that ioglycamide also reaches a higher concentration in the bile when it is administered by slow infusion (Bell *et al.* 1975). In the rhesus monkey the peak concentration is sustained longer with an infusion lasting two hours than one lasting 36 minutes when the same quantity of ioglycamide is administered (Whitney & Bell 1976). The authors' method of choice is to infuse 100 ml of ioglycamide over a period of one hour.

Very precise radiographic technique is essential (Bryan 1971), the most important factors being a low kilovoltage (50–60 Kv), an adequate milliampere/second factor, the avoidance of respiratory blur and accurate positioning, centring and collimation.

Films should be taken at the end of the infusion and at 15 minute intervals thereafter. Once the bile ducts are visualized tomography or zonography should be used. It has been suggested by Burgener & Fischer (1975) that in hepatocellular and obstructive jaundice delayed visualization of the biliary system occurs and films may need to be taken for up to eight hours after the infusion. They state that prolonging the infusion time to six hours does not improve the result, or increase the bile iodine concentration.

In cases where the gallbladder opacifies, it should be examined as in oral cholecystography with views taken in the erect position and after fat.

References

Bauer K., Tragl K. H., Bauer G., Vyeudilik W. & Hocker P. (1974) *Wien. klin. Wschr.*, **86**, 766

Bell G. D., Fayadh M. H., Frank J., Smith P. L. C. & Kelsey-Fry I. (1975) *Gut*, **16**, 841

Bryan G. (1971) *X-Ray Focus*, **11**, 15

Burgener F. A. & Fischer H. W. (1975) *Lancet*, **i**, 274

Darnborough A. & Geffen N. (1966) *Brit. J. Radiol.*, **39**, 827

Finby N. & Blasberg G. (1964) *Gastroenterology*, **46**, 276

Fischer H. W. (1965) *Radiology*, **84**, 483

Foy R. E. (1968) *Radiology*, **90**, 576

Han S. Y., Collins L. C. & Wright R. M. (1969) *Clin Radiol.*, **20**, 332

Jones C. A. & Olbourne N. A. (1973) *Brit. J. Radiol.*, **46**, 711

Kreel L. (1973) *Clin. Gastroent.*, **2**, 185

Lasser E. C., Farr R. S., Fujimagari T. & Tripp W. N. (1962) *Amer. J. Roentgenol.*, **87**, 338

Martinez L. O., Viamonte M., Gassman P. & Boudet L. (1971) *Amer. J. Roentgenol.*, **113**, 10

McNulty J. G. (1968) *Radiology*, **90**, 570

Nolan D. J. & Gibson M. J. (1970) *Brit. J. Radiol.*, **43**, 652

Rosati G. & Schiantarelli P. (1970) *Invest. Radiol.*, **5**, 232

Sargent E. N., Schulman A., Meyers H. I., Gutler R. B., Nicoloff J. T. & DiFazio L. T. (1975) *Amer. J. Roentgenol.*, **125**, 251

Spent J., Spooner R. & Powell L. W. (1969) *Med. J. Aust.*, **2**, 446

Whitney B. P. & Bell C. D. (1972) *Brit. J. Radiol.*, **45**, 891

Whitney B. P. & Bell C. D. (1976) *Brit. J. Radiol.*, **49**, 118

Wise R. E. (1966) *Radiol. Clin. N. Amer.*, **4**, 521

Wise R. E. (1967) *Postgrad. Med.*, **41**, 113

Endoscopic retrograde cholangio-pancreatography (ERCP)

Pancreatography and cholangiography can now be performed as a combined procedure on the same patient by a per-oral technique. A few years ago this would not have seemed possible, but it has been made so by a number of developments resulting from the introduction of fibre-optic endoscopy (Hirschowitz *et al.* 1958). Although in the 1960s Japanese developments were directed towards the production of duodenoscopes, it was not until 1968 that the Machida Company developed a suitable instrument, based on the American Hirschowitz, Rider and Eder fibre-optic endoscopes, and reports began to appear showing the clinical value of this technique (Takagi *et al.* 1970). Endoscopic visualization of the papilla of Vater was described by Watson (1966), whilst McCune *et al.* (1968) were the first to perform endoscopic cannulation of the papilla of Vater employing a modified Eder fibre-optic endoscope. Endoscopic cholangio-pancreatography was described by Oi in 1970, and numerous reports appeared in the Japanese literature to be followed by several European and British papers (Salmon *et al.* 1972; Cotton 1972; Blumgart *et al.* 1972; Burwood *et al.* 1973; Blumgart *et al.* 1974; Salmon 1975).

Indications Endoscopic retrograde cholangio-pancreatography is indicated in the investigation of
1 suspected duodenal pathology;
2 jaundice—persistent undiagnosed jaundice, recurrent undiagnosed jaundice;
3 biliary tract problems—undiagnosed upper abdominal pain (suspected to be biliary in origin); and
4 pancreatic disease—undiagnosed abdominal pain (suspected to be pancreatic in origin), relapsing pancreatitis (diagnosis and assessment), post-operative assessment.

One of the major advantages of retrograde cholangio-pancreatography is the ease with which endoscopic inspection and biopsy prior to filling the pancreatic and bile ducts with contrast medium can be performed; the pylorus, duodenal bulb and duodenal loop can be inspected, although the fourth part of the duodenum cannot usually be reached. Peri-ampullary carcinoma can be excluded by inspection, brush cytology and multiple biopsy and an impacted gallstone may be seen or debris may be found lying in the duodenal lumen, which indicate choledocholithiasis. Other pathology such as gastro-duodenal Crohn's disease, lymphomas and duodenitis, may also be diagnosed in a similar manner.

In the presence of jaundice with serum bilirubin levels in excess of 45 m mol/l or in the presence of impaired hepatic function, intravenous cholangiography may fail to demonstrate the bile ducts and retrograde cholangiography gives the opportunity for making a diagnosis. When it is available endoscopic cholangiography should be performed prior to percutaneous transhepatic cholangiography since it will provide additional information concerning the gastro-duodenal area and the pancreas. There is no need to delay ERCP in patients with jaundice once viral hepatitis and drug-induced or alcohol-induced jaundice have been excluded. Experience with ERCP in the diagnosis of a persistent jaundice has been encouraging (Kasugai *et al.* 1972; Ogoshi *et al*, 1973; Oi 1973; Salmon *et al.* 1973; Blumgart *et al.* 1974; Tables 1 and 2). There is an overall accuracy of over 70 per cent. in the diagnosis of jaundice and laparotomy may be avoided in patients shown to have a normal biliary tree.

Retrograde cholangiography may be useful in the diagnosis of post-cholecystectomy symptoms and of anatomical anomalies such as a low insertion of the cystic duct and variations of the intrahepatic bile ducts. Endoscopic manometry using a micro-balloon catheter is also feasible.

Table 1 Jaundice: diagnostic value of endoscopy and ERCP (from Blumgart, Salmon & Cotton 1974)

Total number of cases	146	
Examined by endoscopy/ERCP	145	
Duodenum entered	144	
Papilla seen	140	
Papilla cannulated	116	(80%)
Diagnostic information		
ERCP	102 ⎫	(75%)
Endoscopy (+ biopsy)	7 ⎭	
Useful information		
Endoscopy	11	(8%)
No diagnostic information	24 ⎫	
Misleading information	⎬	(17%)
Endoscopy	1 ⎭	

Table 2 Jaundice: diagnosis by endoscopy and ERCP (from Blumgart, Salmon & Cotton 1974)

By means of ERCP	
Gallstones	31
Pancreatic or bile duct cancer	25
Sclerosing cholangitis	5
Post-operative stricture	8
Abnormalities of gallbladder	7
Miscellaneous:	
Dilated duct	1
(post-cholecystectomy)	
Debris in dilated duct	1
(post-sphincterotomy)	
Hydatid cyst	1
Tuberculous abscess	1
Normal ducts	22
Endoscopic diagnosis (biopsy positive)	
Ampullary carcinoma	3
Pancreatic carcinoma	2
Gastric carcinoma	1
Stomal ulcer	1
Total	109
Useful information on endoscopy	
Distorted duodenum	11
(probably pancreatic cancer)	

The ability to perform pancreatography in the lightly sedated patient offers the possibility of studying inflammatory and neoplastic disease of the pancreas. The problem of selecting patients with pancreatic cancer at an early enough stage to offer some form of cure, and the differential diagnosis between pancreatitis and carcinoma of the pancreas, are under study at the present time.

The techniques required for cholangio-pancreatography are both endoscopic and radiographic. Endoscopic techniques are difficult and considerable expertise is required, but trained endoscopists throughout the world have demonstrated a consistently high success rate of more than 90 per cent. The various techniques have been described by Cotton *et al.* (1972), Salmon *et al.* (1972), Blumgart & Salmon (1974) Salmon (1974) and Cotton & Salmon (1976).

Method The patient is generally prepared with intravenous diazepam at the time of the examination and is intubated in the left lateral position using a side-viewing duodenoscope. The instrument is positioned in the second part of the duodenum following initial inspection of the pyloric antrum, pylorus and duodenal bulb. It is important to examine the second part of the duodenum, looking particularly for extrinsic compression of the medial wall, encroachment and ulceration of the peri-ampullary region, evidence of peri-ampullary carcinoma, papillitis and duodenal diverticula.

Cannulation Having established the position of the papilla of Vater on the postero-medial wall, a medical ileus is obtained, usually with intravenous hyoscine-N-butyl bromide (Buscopan) or glucagon and a suitable anti-foam agent (e.g. polydimethylsiloxane) may be employed at this time. When the papilla of Vater is in an *en face* position, the patient is usually placed prone, which allows radiography with an undercouch tube.

A polythene catheter (5 French gauge) is then advanced down the instrument channel of the endoscope into the field of view using the instrument-raising bridge and is manipulated into the papillary orifice. It is important to pre-fill the catheter with a suitable contrast medium such as Angiografin 65 per cent. Having cannulated the papilla, contrast medium is then injected under image intensification control. If the biliary system fills first, the contrast medium is changed to a more diluted form such as 25 per cent. Hypaque. Selective cannulation of the bile duct or pancreatic duct is a practical procedure and involves the pre-positioning of both the instrument and the catheter so that the entry of the catheter into the papilla is at right angles to the medial wall when pancreatic duct filling is desired, and parallel to the medial wall with the tip pointing upwards when bile duct filling is desired.

It is important to prevent the injection of air bubbles during contrast filling of the bile or pancreatic duct, and also to know the degree of insertion of the catheter tip, and for this reason 2-mm calibration marks are provided on most of the available catheters. Where a short common channel is present it is clear that insertion of more than 4 mm will only result in contrast filling of one duct, whereas a 2-mm insertion would be more likely to fill both ducts simultaneously.

Excessive duodenal motility Assuming that the instrument has been advanced correctly into the second part of the duodenum, initial problems may be involved with excessive motility, bubbles and frothing from bile, or the papilla of Vater

is difficult to identify. The usual reason for initial excess motility is either anxiety on the part of the patient or the excessive use of air insufflation. If after a few minutes the motility has not ceased on its own it will be necessary to use an anti-cholinergic agent at this stage, although normally it is best to use this agent only at the last minute because of the relatively short duration of its action.

Finding the papilla Duodenal diverticula usually appear near the papilla of Vater, so that when these are noted the position of the papilla may be located. In a few cases the papilla actually lies within a diverticulum and may not be accessible for cannulation. In cases where it cannot be identified, the endoscope has usually been passed beyond the papilla in which case the endoscopist should withdraw it slowly up the medial wall, identify each circular fold and look for the landmarks of the papilla, namely longitudinal folds passing up the medial wall. These folds converge on the papilla which may lie under a transverse fold and in this case the catheter may have to be advanced in order to lift up a transverse fold and demonstrate the papilla underneath. Occasionally a rudimentary or flat papilla may be difficult to identify. It should be noted that an accessory papilla is very often present but lies more anteriorly and about one centimetre proximal to the main papilla of Vater. A special problem is posed following a Polya-type partial gastrectomy. In this instance the technique is fundamentally different since one is approaching the papilla of Vater upstream in an afferent loop. For this reason a forward-viewing endoscope such as a paediatric gastro-duodenoscope may well be necessary to perform cannulation. Fortunately these cases are rare, but success has been reported (Sáfrány 1972).

Injection of contrast medium In the majority of cases pancreatic duct filling occurs first; in nearly every case it is advantageous to obtain filling of both systems, since not only may primary biliary disease give rise to pancreatitis but primary pancreatic disease—whether inflammatory or neoplastic—may involve the biliary tract, and knowledge of this may influence the patient's management. When filling the pancreatic duct, it is important to get side branch filling, filling of the uncinate lobe branch, and filling to the tail. Excessive parenchymal filling should be avoided. It is important to obtain pictures after removal of the endoscope, but only after a short delay, since rapid emptying may otherwise occur. Small lesions may be missed if they lie behind the endoscope. The use of a videotape recorder, delayed films, sequential radiographs and cine-radiography may all aid in obtaining dynamic data of sphincter of Oddi function and the dynamics of duct filling and emptying.

It is important to recognize when contrast medium is filling a pancreatic cyst because of the danger of stasis and abscess formation. When this occurs, the examination should be terminated and either surgery performed or the cyst assessed

by a less invasive technique such as ultrasound. Filling of ducts in the pancreatic head alone may be due to the tip of the catheter becoming wedged in a branch of the main pancreatic duct, a persistent ventral pancreas, or an organic obstruction due to either an inflammatory stricture or to carcinoma. Radiographs of the filled pancreatic duct are taken in the straight and oblique positions and then again with the patient prone and supine following withdrawal of the endoscope. A lateral film with the patient lying on the left side is also useful. Delayed screening at five minutes is performed to monitor duct emptying. During bile duct filling, the contrast medium is changed to 25 per cent. Hypaque. The amount of contrast medium injected will depend on the capacity of the biliary tree and the information that is being obtained. Filling of the intrahepatic ducts is usually achieved with the patient lying as flat as possible for if he is on his left side, the right lobe ducts tend to empty. It is unwise to inject too much contrast medium above an incomplete obstruction, as this can be retained and provoke a chemical cholangitis which may then be superseded by infection. Since the biliary tree retains contrast medium better than the pancreatic duct, adequate undercouch and overcouch radiographs can be performed following withdrawal of the endoscope. Oblique and coned views in the prone, supine and upright positions are performed to delineate calculi in the main ducts and the gallbladder.

Pure pancreatic juice collection is now possible following selective pancreatic duct cannulation, and pure juice cytology following a body-weight dose of secretin is of particular value. It seems at the present time that pure juice should be collected at 0, 5 and 10 minutes and subjected as rapidly as possible—and certainly within four hours—to cytocentrifugation and fixation. Interpretation of normal pancreatic cells requires considerable skill, but current literature suggests that this additional information may aid in the differential diagnosis of pancreatic carcinoma (Hatfield *et al.* 1974).

Table 3 A survey of endoscopic retrograde cholangio-pancreatography experience in the United States (Bilbao *et al.* 1976)

		%
Endoscope owners queried	402	
Answers returned	222	55
Total reported ERCPs	10,435	
Reported 'successes'	7,304	70
Detailed reports	8,681	
Complications	270	3
Fatal complications	15	0·2

Complications Endoscopic cholangio-pancreatography is essentially a safe procedure, but there are a number of hazards that should be taken into account. A recent survey of 10,435 examinations (Bilbao *et al.* 1976) showed a procedural failure in 30 per cent., 15 per cent. with

Table 4 Analysis of complications from ERCP survey depicted in Table 3 (Bilbao *et al.* 1976)

ERCP	Complications	Incidence	Deaths	Fatality rate
		%		%
Injection pancreatitis	94	1·0		
Cholangitic sepsis	72	0·8	8	10
Drug reactions	51	0·6		
Pancreatic sepsis-pseudocyst	25	0·3	5	20
Instrumental injury	16	0·2	2	13
Aspiration pneumonia	8	0·1		
Miscellaneous	4			

'experienced' workers, complications in 3 per cent. and death in 0·2 per cent. (Tables 3 & 4). The chief complications include pancreatitis, cholangitis, pancreatic sepsis, instrumental injury to the gastrointestinal tract and drug reactions. Pancreatitis was invariably associated with injection into the pancreatic duct, and sepsis associated with obstruction or a non-draining pseudocyst. The demonstration of bile duct obstruction or pancreatic pseudocyst is an indication for immediate antibiotic therapy.

References

Bilbao M. K., Dotter C. T., Lee T. G. & Katon R. M. (1976) *Gastroenterology*, **70**, 314

Blumgart L. H. & Salmon P. R. (1974) in *Recent Advances in Surgery*, p.36 (Ed. Taylor S.). Edinburgh: Churchill–Livingstone

Blumgart L. H., Salmon P. & Cotton P. B. (1974) *Surg. Gynec. Obstet.*, **138**, 565

Blumgart L. H., Salmon P., Cotton P. B., Davies G. T., Burwood R., Beales J. S. M., Lawrie B., Skirving A. & Read A. E. (1972) *Lancet*, **ii**, 1269

Burwood R. J., Davies G. T., Lawrie B. W., Blumgart L. H. & Salmon P. R. (1973) *Clin. Radiol.*, **24**, 397

Cotton P. B. (1972) *Gut*, **13**, 1014

Cotton P. B. (1977) *Gut*, **18**, 316

Cotton P. B., Salmon P. R., Blumgart L. H., Burwood R. J., Davies G. T., Lawrie B. W., Pierce J. W. & Read A. E. (1972) *Lancet*, **i**, 53

Cotton P. B. & Salmon P. R. (1976) *Topics in Modern Gastrointestinal Endoscopy*. London: Heinemann Medical

Hatfield A. R. W., Whittaker R. & Gibbs D. D. (1974) *Gut*, **15**, 305

Hirschowitz B. I., Curtiss L. E., Peters C. W. & Pollard H. M. (1958) *Gastroenterology*, **35**, 50

Kasugai T., Kuno N., Kizu M., Kobayashi S. & Hattori K. (1972) *Gastroenterology*, **63**, 227

McCune W. S., Shorb P. E. & Moscovitz H. (1968) *Ann. Surg.*, **167**, 752

Ogoshi K., Niwa M., Hara Y. & Nebel O. T. (1973) *Gastroenterology*, **64**, 210

Oi I. (1970) *Gastrointest. Endosc.*, **17**, 59

Oi I. (1973) In *Endoscopy of the Small Intestine with Retrograde Pancreato-cholangiography*, p.1010 (Ed. Demling L. & Classen M.). Stuttgart: George Thieme

Sáfrány L. (1972) *Endoscopy*, **4**, 198

Salmon P. R. (1974) *Fibre-optic Endoscopy*, London: Pitman Medical

Salmon P. R. (1975) In *Modern Trends in Gastroenterology*, p.231 (Ed. Read A. E.). London: Butterworth

Salmon P. R., Blumgart L., Burwood R. J., Davies G. & Read A. E. (1973) in *Endoscopy of the Small Intestine with Retrograde Pancreato-cholangiography*, p.98 (Ed. Demling L. & Classen M.). Stuttgart: George Thieme

Salmon P. R., Brown P., Htut T. & Read A. E. (1972) *Gut*, **13**, 170

Takagi K., Ikeda S., Nakagawa Y. *et al.* (1970) *Gastroenterology*, **59**, 445

Watson W. C. (1966) *Lancet*, **i**, 902

Percutaneous transhepatic cholangiography

GORDON EVISON

The idea of injecting contrast medium directly into dilated bile ducts had been discussed since the early days of radiology. It received a further impetus in the 1950s when liver biopsy by direct puncture was introduced, but the main objection to the method was the rigidity of the metal needle. With the introduction of flexible polythene catheters, this objection was largely overcome and a technique was described from the Royal Free Hospital, London (Shaldon 1962), which forms the basis of a practical and widely accepted examination.

Indications The major indication for conventional percutaneous transhepatic cholangiography is undiagnosed jaundice which is believed to be due to extrahepatic obstruction and associated with dilated intrahepatic bile ducts. Facilities for prompt surgical relief of biliary obstruction should be available. Percutaneous cholangiography may also be used to assess the proximal bile ducts for surgery where the cause of obstruction is already known. Fine-needle cholangiography has broadened these indications: as normal calibre ducts may be entered, jaundiced patients can be investigated earlier before the bile ducts have had time to become dilated, and the biliary systems of patients with primary biliary cirrhosis and sclerosing cholangitis may be outlined.

Contraindications A tendency to bleeding, sensitivity to contrast agents and evidence of cholangitis are contraindications to percutaneous cholangiography. Liver scintiscanning and ultrasound may demonstrate liver metastases which make puncture difficult and suggest that the procedure is unnecessary.

Method The patient, whose prothrombin time must be within normal limits (BSR < 1·3), is premedicated on the ward half an hour before the examination. Further sedation may be given before or during the procedure, intravenous diazepam being very useful. The examination is carried out in the X-ray department on a standard tilting screening table, using image intensification.

Sheathed needle After preliminary skin preparation, a fine polythene tube is introduced on a long 20-gauge needle directly through the skin into the liver. An anterior sub-costal approach, 1 cm below and to the right of the xiphisternum, is commonly used, but some workers prefer a lateral intercostal route. Thorough infiltration with local anaesthetic prior to puncture is essential, and opening up a wide track through the tissue planes using mosquito forceps is recommended. The tube and needle are inserted deep into the liver and the needle removed at once, leaving the flexible tube in position. This is gradually withdrawn until bile is aspirated, indicating that the tip of the tube is in a bile duct. Contrast medium is then injected, under screen control, the amount necessary to fill the biliary tree varying from 30 ml to 120 ml. The screening table may be tilted to aid filling, but it is wise not to rotate the patient too much as the hold on the bile duct by the tube is often precarious. Spot films are exposed to show detail of individual areas. At the end of the procedure the tube is left in position for drainage until laparotomy, which should follow within six hours.

Fine needle A recent development has been a return to the use of a fine metal needle with an outer diameter of 0·7 mm which is extremely flexible (Okuda *et al.* 1974). A lateral intercostal approach with puncture in the mid-axillary line is used. Contrast medium is injected as the needle is withdrawn until a bile duct is outlined. Excessive parenchymal injection should be avoided, and blood vessels are easily recognized as the medium within them is soon washed away. Five or six punctures at different angles or sites are possible. Meglumine iothalamate (280 mg iodine/ml) seems to be an adequate contrast agent and 20–30 ml is usually enough to outline the biliary tree.

The advantages of this method are that it is possible to enter bile ducts that are not significantly dilated so that jaundiced patients may be investigated earlier and normal biliary systems may be visualized. If an obstructed biliary system is outlined we believe immediate surgical decompression is indicated, as with the conventional technique; alternatively the puncture may be repeated using a sheathed needle so as to leave a catheter for drainage.

The transjugular approach is another recent development (Hanafee & Weiner 1967). The right internal jugular vein is catheterized by the Seldinger technique and the catheter advanced through the vena cavae into the hepatic vein. A modified Ross trans-septal needle is then used to puncture the liver parenchyma and adjacent bile duct. The quoted advantages of this technique are the avoidance of peritoneal bleeding and bile leakage.

Complications Bile leakage, bleeding, acute cholangitis and septicaemia are the important complications of the percutaneous techniques. Leaving a drainage catheter *in situ* until operation helps to decompress the biliary system. Though bile leakage and bleeding are less frequent and severe if the fine-needle technique is used, these complications do occur and immediate laparotomy and decompression may still be necessary. Acute cholangitis and septicaemia may occur with the fine needle and catheter techniques, and though more common in association with gallstones they may occur in neoplastic obstruction, so that antibiotic cover is indicated if an obstructive lesion is suspected. The overall complication rate for fine needle cholangiography is about 7·5 per cent (Okuda *et al.* 1974), which is similar to that for the sheathed needle technique (Elias 1976).

References

Elias E. (1976) *Gut,* **17,** 801

Hanafee W. & Weiner M. (1967) *Radiology*, **88**, 35

Okuda K., Tanikawa K., Emura T. *et al.* (1974) *Amer. J. dig. Dis.*, **19**, 21

Shaldon S. (1962) *Proc. roy. Soc. Med.*, **55**, 587

Operative cholangiography

Operative cholangiography might be considered as part of the surgical exploration of the bile duct and has been recommended as a routine procedure in all patients undergoing cholecystectomy or bile duct surgery (George 1973). The investigation can be used to demonstrate or confirm the presence of common duct calculi, to delineate anomalous ducts and biliary strictures and may also be used to demonstrate lesions involving the intrahepatic bile ducts such as neoplasms and cystic dilatation (Caroli 1973).

Method The cystic duct may be cannulated with a fine catheter, pre-filled with saline to avoid the injection of air bubbles which may be mistaken for calculi. Dilute solutions (150 mg iodine/ml) of contrast medium such as Hypaque 25 per cent. or Urografin 30 per cent. (145 mg iodine/ml) are injected so as to reveal small calculi which would be obscured by denser concentrations of contrast agent. An initial film taken after 4–5 ml and another after 10–15 ml are usually adequate. Better views are obtained if the contrast medium is injected during the exposure. A lead screen for the operator is mandatory. One of the major problems of operative radiography is the low power of the portable equipment which has to be used, but this disadvantage is offset by the ability to suspend patient movement and compensate with longer exposure times.

Gridded film cassettes are used to reduce scattered radiation from the patient and so to improve the diagnostic quality of the film. The transverse axis of a gridded cassette must be at right angles to the axis of the incident X-ray beam. Many surgical texts suggest that the surgical table and its film cassette tunnel should be angled 15 degrees to throw the bile duct away from the overlying spine. As it is impossible to obtain an adequate radiograph in these circumstances with the grid lines not parallel to the X-ray beam the cassette should be inserted sideways under the patient so that the grid lines lie across. It is easier to angle the X-ray beam rather than the patient, operating table and film.

Le Quesne (1960) lists the criteria for a normal operative cholangiogram as follows
1 the calibre of the common bile duct is 12 mm or less;
2 there is free flow of contrast medium into the duodenum;
3 the terminal narrow segment of the duct is clearly seen on at least one film;
4 no filling defects are present; and
5 there is no excess retrograde filling of the hepatic ducts.

If there is doubt about the appearances on the initial films these should be repeated with straight and oblique views taken during filling with contrast medium. Screening with a mobile image intensifer is no alternative to a good film technique since the resolution of this method is very poor and calculi may be missed.

T-tube cholangiography is similar to the operative technique in that air bubbles in the biliary tree must be avoided. Clamping the T-tube as close to the patient as possible and using a pre-filled contrast injecting system are important. This examination is usually of better quality and easier to perform since more powerful equipment is available in the X-ray department. Similar amounts of dilute contrast medium and similar radiographic views are used as for operative cholangiography.

References

Caroli J. (1973) *Clin. Gastroent.*, **2**, 147

George P. (1973) *Clin. Gastroent.*, **2**, 127

Le Quesne L. P. (1960) *Proc. roy. Soc. Med.*, **53**, 852

Hepatic, biliary and pancreatic scintigraphy

E. R. DAVIES

Colloid scintigraphy Colloid particles less than $0.5\ \mu m$ in size are taken up by the reticulo-endothelial cells where they remain physiologically inert. In a normal adult about 85 per cent. of injected colloidal particles are accumulated in the liver, with most of the remainder accumulated in the spleen, and a very small number in the bone marrow and lymph nodes. The compound of choice is $^{99}Tc^{m}$-sulphur colloid, with $^{113}I^{m}$ colloid as an acceptable alternative. An activity of 1–2 mCi is injected intravenously and scanning can begin within a few minutes. The Gamma camera is the most satisfactory instrument because it enables the examination to be finished quickly. It is customary to do anterior, lateral and posterior images of the liver, as well as at least two views of the spleen. The anterior and posterior images of the liver are roughly triangular but the shape of the lateral image is more rounded and more variable. The activity within the liver is homogeneous apart from a recognized band of low activity between the right and left lobes. On the lower margin of the anterior image there is an impression at the porta hepatis, and another impression just lateral to this due to the gallbladder. Occasionally the gallbladder is intrahepatic and this produces a circumscribed defect within the anterior image. The size of the liver varies with the size of the individual but there is no constant relationship with the body height, mass or surface area. Normal variation in liver shapes such as Riedel's lobe can be recognized easily. The commonest cause of variations in position is an alteration in the level of the right dome of the diaphragm, and the normal respiratory movement of the diaphragm is enough to cause some irregularity in the upper surface of the liver.

131I Rose Bengal scanning   Rose Bengal is cleared from the blood by the hepatocytes and because of the very rich blood supply to the liver, the blood clearance is rapid, with a half time of approximately 15 minutes. Images of the liver may be obtained between 15 and 30 minutes after intravenous injection of 150–250 μCi of labelled Rose Bengal, and in the normal subject some activity may already be present in the gallbladder, or even in the gut, by this stage. The study is designed to record the excretion of activity from the liver into the gut, and therefore the patency of the biliary tree. Although liver architecture may be visualized with this compound, count rates are low and small bowel activity tends to obscure the outline of the liver. Anterior images are taken of the upper abdomen 30 minutes and 60 minutes after injection; activity seen in the gut during this time indicates a normally patent biliary tree. It is usually unnecessary to give a fat meal or intravenous cholecystokinin to ensure gallbladder contraction. Delay in intestinal activity indicates some degree of cholestasis or obstruction and further images should then be taken at 6, 24, 48 and 96 hours. In the presence of obstruction there is insufficient activity in the gut to be recognized even at 96 hours, but in the presence of cholestasis there is usually sufficient activity to be recognized during the late images (Davies *et al.* 1976).

In the presence of biliary obstruction, a small quantity of Rose Bengal may be observed in the renal areas. It is important not to confuse this with intestinal activity and this is done by noting the position and constancy of the activity in serial scans.

Isotope cholecystography   Radiographic study of gallbladder emptying is unacceptable because of the high radiation dose involved in protracted cine filming or multiple serial films. The use of a radioactive tracer that is accumulated in the gallbladder has obvious advantages and several compounds have been advocated. The following is a simple technique that requires only the oral administration of 10 μCi of 131I sodium ipodate solution. This compound is given on the evening before the examination and on the next morning the test is done on the fasting patient. A collimated scintillation counter is suspended vertically over the area of maximal radioactivity and its position over the skin marked in case the patient subsequently changes position. The count rate is monitored by a pen recorder, which provides a continuous trace of changes throughout the examination. Gallbladder emptying is stimulated either by giving cholecystokinin intravenously or a cholagogue orally. A suitable stimulus is a flavoured emulsion containing 20 ml arachis oil. It can be shown that the rate at which the count-rate falls is proportional to the rate of contraction of the gallbladder. Several components of contraction have been described, but it is extremely difficult to assess more than the overall contraction rate from a simple tracing. Activity does not fall to zero during the examination because there is some background activity from the liver and adjacent bowel.

However, the technique offers a convenient way of studying gallbladder emptying in a variety of disease conditions (Chapple *et al.* 1975).

Pancreatic scanning   There is no ideal compound for pancreatic scanning but that most widely used is 75Se-selenomethionine. This compound follows the distribution of methionine in the body and therefore is accumulated in the pancreas because of enzyme synthesis, and in the liver because of protein metabolism. Some activity may be found in the thyroid gland because of hormone synthesis. The most important activity is in the liver, which may obscure the outline of the pancreas, particularly if it is large or overlies the pancreas. For this reason it is customary to do a liver scan immediately before doing the pancreas scan. This image can be used for visual or electronic subtraction from the final image in order to obtain the true pancreatic image. Many techniques have been suggested to enhance pancreatic accumulation of radioactivity but none is satisfactory.

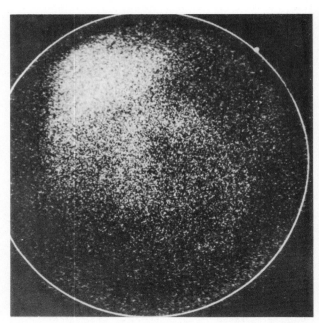

2.1   **Normal pancreatic function**   *Pancreatic scintiscan* (75Se-selenomethionine scan in the anterior position recorded on a gamma camera)   Pancreatic uptake is seen as an ⌐ shaped area of activity in the centre of the scan, which lies below and to the left of the liver, which also shows activity

The examination is usually begun immediately after the patient has had a meal. A preliminary liver scan is followed by intravenous injection of 100–150 μCi 75Se-selenomethionine and the patient is given a glass of Complan to drink. Pancreatic images are taken immediately using a Gamma camera with its crystal tilted 10 degrees towards the head of the patient. It is advisable to take as many images as possible during the first hour after injection as pancreatic accumulation depends on enzyme synthesis in the pancreas and this does not occur evenly throughout the pancreas. Therefore it is important to record the sequence of activity through the pancreas on three or four images. The normal pancreas runs obliquely or horizontally across the upper abdomen. A variety of shapes has been described but some of these are the result of amalgamation of pancreatic image with radioactivity in the duodeno-jejunal flexure. This may be just above or below the body of the pancreas, thereby giving the image either a sigmoid or horseshoe shape.

The commonest abnormality of pancreatic image is absence of activity which may be due to a tumour in the pancreas or to acute pancreatitis or relapsing pancreatitis. The distinction between these conditions cannot be made from the scan at the moment (Agnew *et al.* 1976). Diminished activity may occur in chronic pancreatitis and pancreatic calculi, but can also accompany diabetes mellitus, fibrocystic disease and congenital failure of exocrine function. Unfortunately

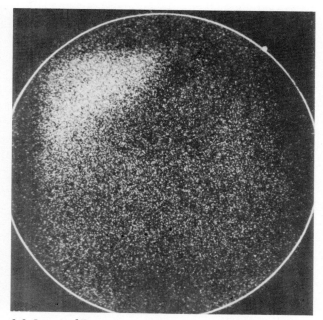

2.2 Impaired Pancreatic uptake *Pancreatic scintiscan* Very little activity is evident in the region of the pancreas although the liver uptake is normal

activity may be diminished by some extra-pancreatic diseases such as carcinoma elsewhere in the body, severe general ill health and advancing years. Localized deficiency in activity is usually the result of carcinoma in the pancreas though it may also be caused by penetrating gastric ulcer, para-pancreatic cysts, operation on the upper abdomen such as gastrectomy and vagotomy, and arterial aneurysm. Increased uptake by the normal or diseased pancreas is exceptionally rare and

difficult to evaluate though it has been recorded, and exceptionally in anaplastic primary carcinoma of the pancreas. On rare occasions pseudo-pancreatic cysts have been shown to have increased uptake, as has carcinoma extending outside the pancreas.

References

Agnew J. E., Maze M. & Mitchell C. J. (1976) *Brit. J. Radiol.*, **49**, 979

Chapple M. J., Nolan D. J., Low-Beer T. S. & Davies E. R. (1975) *Brit. J. Radiol.*, **48**, 19

Davies E. R., Morris J. N., Read A. E. & Powell N. (1976) *Clin. Radiol.*, **27**, 227

Ultrasound examination

F. G. M. ROSS

By the use of ultrasound it is possible to demonstrate the gallbladder in most patients and also the intra- and extrahepatic bile ducts, when they are dilated. Thus the liver and the upper abdomen down to the level of the head of the pancreas must be examined. The use of grey-scale instruments has improved the quality of biliary and pancreatic ultrasound in recent years, and technical improvements are still being made.

Indications Ultrasound is of value in the examination of the biliary system in patients in whom radiological examination has failed or is impossible, or in order to try to enhance the information already obtained by other methods. It is also of value in patients in whom the use of X-radiation is undesirable, such as pregnant women. Its greatest use is in patients with suspected gallbladder disease who show no opacification of the gallbladder at oral cholecystography and in patients with jaundice which may be due to intrahepatic or extrahepatic bile duct obstruction. Calculi may be shown within the biliary tree or tumours arising in the pancreas may be evident.

Method The patient should fast for at least 12 hours before the examination in order that the gallbladder should be at its maximum size at the time of the examination. The factor that limits ultrasonic examination of the abdomen is gas in the bowel. The gas produces an impenetrable barrier to the ultrasonic beam and gives artefacts due to reverberation.

Various methods have been tried to overcome the adverse effects of gas in the stomach, such as aspirating the gas by stomach tube or filling the stomach with water. These have not proved to be very successful. Some benefit may be obtained by use of Simethicone tablets for two days before the examination (Summer & Filly 1977).

The patient is examined in the supine position and the scans

are made during suspended respiration. In most patients the best demonstration of the liver and biliary tract is obtained on inspiration. Transverse and longitudinal scans are made as a routine. The transverse scans are taken from just below the xiphisternum at 1-cm intervals down as far as is necessary to make certain that the lower end of the common bile duct has been included. A good guide to this is just below the origin of the superior mesenteric artery from the aorta, a part which can frequently be defined. Longitudinal scans are also made at 1-cm intervals as far as is necessary on each side of the midline to ensure adequate coverage of the biliary tree. In order to define the long axis of the gallbladder its position is obtained from the transverse scans. The apparatus is then positioned so that an oblique scan is made along the length of the gallbladder after marking this line on the skin. Finally scans at right angles to the long axis may be made to define the gallbladder's true diameter (Holm et al. 1976). Scans at high and low gain setting should be obtained in order best to differentiate the gallbladder from its surrounding tissues and in order to be certain to reveal any echogenic masses within its lumen. The technique of linear section scanning should be used and compounding kept to a minimum. Angular subcostal scans parallel to the right costal margin may also be very informative.

References

Holm H. H., Kristensen J. K., Rasmussen S. N., Pedersen J. F. & Hancke S. (1976) *Abdominal Ultrasound*. p.76. Copenhagen: Munksgaard

Summer G. & Filly R. A. (1977) *J. clin. Ultrasound*, **5**, 87

Computed tomography

Computed tomography has become established as a major advance in the visualization of tissue structures and the initial success with the EMI cranial scanner which was introduced in 1972 has prompted the development of whole-body scanners. The examination of body sections presents widely differing problems such as respiratory, cardiovascular or peristaltic movements and the variations in patient size and tissue density. Using fast scanning cycles and more powerful computers these difficulties have been partially overcome and images with a high degree of definition can be produced.

The basic system comprises a scanning gantry which surrounds the patient couch and a computer with control, viewing and data storage facilities. The gantry contains the X-ray tube and an array of highly sensitive detectors which are located opposite the tube on the scanning frame. A collimated X-ray beam 13 mm wide is used and the photons in the emergent beam are measured by the detectors after they have passed through the patient. The scan of a single transverse, 13 mm wide slice can be completed within 20 seconds during which time 300,000 readings from the detectors are digitalized and fed to the computer which is then able to calculate the X-ray absorption values of tissues throughout the slice. The resulting image is such that individual picture elements of 1·5 mm × 1·5 mm can be resolved.

Computed tomography has the advantage that good tissue resolution can be achieved without the need for invasive techniques and is acceptable to most patients who are able to hold their breath for 20 seconds and who can lie flat for 30 minutes or so. Unfortunately, it is expensive and available only in the largest centres, but it is likely that in time costs will begin to fall, so that units will be available in most district hospitals.

Experience with computed tomography of patients with biliary and pancreatic disease is very recent but seems to be encouraging (Haaga *et al.* 1976). Pancreatic lesions may produce evidence of gland enlargement or mass, obliteration of the peripancreatic or perivascular fat planes, and widening of the bile ducts due to biliary obstruction. Comparisons with ultrasound investigations suggest that it is more reliable in the demonstration of pancreatic abnormalities (Cotton *et al.* 1977); however ultrasonography is undergoing technical improvement, is cheaper to buy and may also be amenable to computer techniques. Bile duct dilatation and calculi are evident with both methods, although either technique may sometimes fail to show metastases in the liver because these have the same radiodensity or the same echogenicity as surrounding normal tissue.

References

Cotton P. B., Denyer M. E., Husband J., Meire H. B. & Kreel L. (1977) *Gut*, **18**, 399

Haaga J. R., Alfidi R. J., Zelch M. G., Meary T. F., Boller M., Gonzalez L. & Jelden G. L. (1976) *Radiology*, **120**, 589

Kreel L. Ed. (1978) *Medical Imaging: a Basic Course*. Aylesbury: HM+ M Publishers

The anatomy of the intrahepatic bile ducts

The liver consists of two major lobes which are divided by the lobar or main boundary fissure, which, on the visceral aspect of the liver, passes through the gallbladder fossa and the fossa for the inferior vena cava. There is no indication of the lobar fissure on the parietal surface of the liver, though it lies well to the right of the attachment of the falciform ligament. The trunk of the middle hepatic vein runs within this fissure and no branches of the bile ducts, hepatic artery or portal vein cross this fissure except in the region of the porta hepatis (Healey & Schroy 1953). Each lobe is divided into two segments by fissures which are evident on casts. The right lobe is divided by an oblique fissure which passes from the postero-superior aspect to the lower border of the liver anteriorly and extends to the porta hepatis. The ventro-cranial segment of the right lobe is called the anterior segment and the dorso-caudal segment is called the posterior segment.

A comparable fissure divides the left lobe into medial and lateral segments and lies approximately in the position of the insertion of the falciform ligament. The medial segment corresponds in part to the quadrate lobe. The caudate lobe cannot be included in either right or left lobes of the liver as its duct drainage is variable. It is situated on the posterior aspect of the liver and can be divided into right and left portions and the caudate process which lies between the porta hepatis and the fossa for the inferior vena cava. Each of the four major liver segments may be divided in accord with their biliary drainage into two areas—superior and inferior.

The intrahepatic duct anatomy of the human liver has been studied in post-mortem specimens both radiologically and by corrosion techniques (Hjortsjo 1951; Healey & Schroy 1953). The nomenclature adopted here is that suggested by Healey & Schroy and is the one commonly used in Great Britain and the United States.

The bile duct system starts at the cellular level where canaliculi without endothelial lining form a network of channels between the liver cells. From the canaliculi bile passes into endothelialized intralobular ductules, interlobular and then septal ductules; these unite to form branches of the segmental ducts which join to form the two main hepatic ducts that emerge from the liver at the porta hepatis. In cross section, bile ducts have an elliptical form and are accompanied by hepatic artery branches and portal vein distributaries which show a similar pattern of branching within the liver. The hepatic artery branch usually lies behind the segmental bile duct and the portal vein branch.

Biliary drainage of the right lobe In each of the ninety-seven cases studied by Healey & Schroy, two ducts drained this lobe—one from the anterior segment and one from the posterior segment. The latter is longer and superior in position to the anterior duct and they both receive branches from the superior and inferior areas of the two main segments. In 83 per cent. of specimens the posterior segment duct received the posterior inferior area duct. Aberrant drainage of the superior or inferior area ducts of the anterior segment was observed in 20 per cent. of specimens and in each the abnormal duct drained into the posterior segment duct.

In 72 per cent. of specimens the right segmental ducts united to form

3 The Anatomy of the Bile Ducts

the right hepatic duct: in 22 per cent. the right posterior segment duct extended to the left of the lobar fissure to enter the left hepatic duct, and in 6 per cent. the right anterior segment duct extended to the left of the lobar fissure to enter the left hepatic duct.

A subvesical duct in the bed of the gallbladder but which did not connect with it was observed in about one-third of cases.

inferior areas of the medial segment are each drained by two ducts which unite and drain inconstantly. A recognizable left hepatic duct is present in only two-thirds of cases.

Biliary drainage of the caudate lobe The ducts from each of the three portions of the caudate lobe may unite to drain or drain separately into either the right, left or common hepatic ducts.

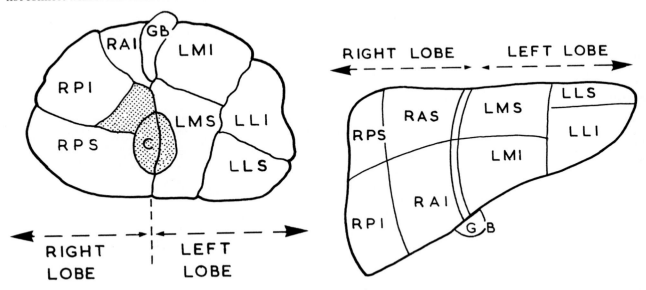

Diagram 3.1—The areas of the liver (L. *inferior aspect;* R. *anterior aspect*)

Key to Diags 3.1–3.3 and Figs 3.1 onwards

c   = caudate lobe ducts
cbd = common bile duct
chd = common hepatic duct
gb = gall bladder
l   = left hepatic duct
lli   = left lateral inferior area duct
lls   = left lateral superior area duct
lmi = left medial inferior area ducts
lms = left medial superior ducts
ra   = right anterior segment duct
rai = right anterior inferior area duct
ras = right anterior superior area duct
r   = right hepatic duct
rp   = right posterior segment duct
rpi   = right posterior inferior area duct
rps = right posterior superior area duct

Biliary drainage of the left lobe The lateral segment is divided into a small superior area and a large inferior area. The inferior area duct is usually longer and larger than the superior area duct, and courses through the lateral segment in an arc which is concave upwards. The superior area duct begins at the upper outer angle of the liver and follows an oblique course towards the porta where it joins the inferior area duct to form the lateral segment duct. The superior and

The anatomy of the extrahepatic bile ducts

The common hepatic duct is formed in the region of the porta hepatis by the junction of the right and left hepatic ducts in about three-quarters of normal subjects. Segmental ducts may join the common hepatic duct directly so that it may be formed by the union of three or more ducts (Healey & Schroy 1953). Anomalous ducts which join the hepatic, cystic or common bile ducts below the porta hepatis are not additional ducts but segmental, usually right-sided, ducts that have united at a lower level than normal. They occur in about 10 per cent. of subjects (Eisendrath 1918; Flint 1923). Undetected injury to anomalous ducts at cholecystectomy may produce a troublesome external biliary fistula or bile peritonitis.

The cystic duct is usually of similar length to the common hepatic duct and they are commonly bound together by fibrous tissues for two or more centimetres before they unite above the upper border of the duodenum. It is usual for the cystic duct to open into the right side of the main bile duct, but there are wide variations in the course, level and site of implantation of the cystic duct which may enter the front, the back or even the left side, taking a spiral course around the main duct (Williams 1962). The cystic duct may join the right hepatic duct or the duodenum directly (Hand 1973).

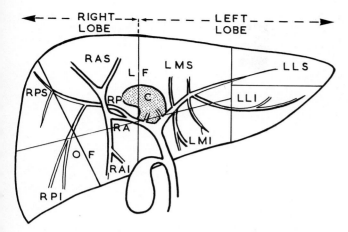

Diag. 3.2 The normal pattern of the intrahepatic bile ducts

The length of the common bile duct varies from 1·5 to 9·0 cm (average 5·0 cm) depending on the type of cystic duct entry. The internal diameter of the common bile duct measured on radiographs above the level of the pancreas averages 5 to 7 mm. There is variation in the agreed upper limit of normal from 10 to 15 mm (Wise & O'Brien 1956; Le Quesne et al. 1959; Mahour et al. 1967). A width of 14 mm or more should be considered abnormal, although in old age it may be greater than this without evidence of obstruction (Kreel et al. 1973). The common hepatic duct is slightly wider than the common bile duct (Dowdy 1962) giving a tapered configuration to the normal main bile duct.

The common bile duct runs in the lesser omentum anterior to the portal vein. It passes behind the first part of the duodenum in a groove in the back of the pancreas to the papilla which lies on the postero-medial wall of the descending duodenum. In two-thirds of cases the bile duct and pancreatic duct join to form a common pancreatico-biliary duct, whilst in a small minority (about 4 per cent.) these ducts are separated at the papilla. In 27 per cent. there is a common septum to the tip of the papilla (Dowdy 1969). Dilatation of the pancreatico-biliary channel to form an ampulla is unusual. The common

bile duct is surrounded by a thickening of longitudinal and circular fibres as it passes through the duodenal wall and the sphincter of Oddi, and the lumen in this region is consequently narrowed. The length of the thickened segment varies from 11 to 27 mm (Hand 1973). The sphincter is normally contracted and can withstand a pressure of 15–25 cm of water in the common bile duct; relaxation is induced by cholecystokinin.

References

Dowdy G. S., Waldron G. W. & Brown W. G. (1962) *Arch. Surg.*, **84**, 229

Dowdy G. S. Jnr. (1969) *The Biliary Tract*. Philadelphia: Lea & Febiger

Eisendrath D. N. (1918) *J. Amer. med. Ass.*, **71**, 864

Flint E. R. (1923) *Brit. J. Surg.*, **10**, 509

Hand B. H. (1973) *Clin. Gastroent.*, **2**, 3

Healey J. E. & Schroy P. C. (1953) *Arch. Surg.*, **66**, 599

Hjortsjo C. H. (1951) *Acta Anat. (Basel)*, **11**, 599

Kreel L., Sandin B. & Slavin G. (1973) *Clin. Radiol.*, **24**, 154

Le Quesne L. P., Whiteside C. G. & Hand B. H. (1959) *Brit. med. J.*, **i**, 329

Mahour G. H., Wakim K. G. & Ferris D. O. (1967) *Ann. Surg.*, **165**, 415

Williams J. E. (1962) *Clin. Radiol.*, **13**, 333

Wise R. E. & O'Brien R. G. (1956) *J. Amer. med. Ass.*, **160**, 819

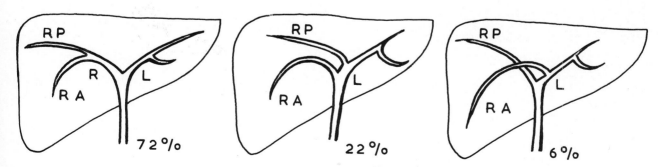

Diag. 3.3. Variations in the drainage of the right segmental ducts (after Healey & Schroy 1953)

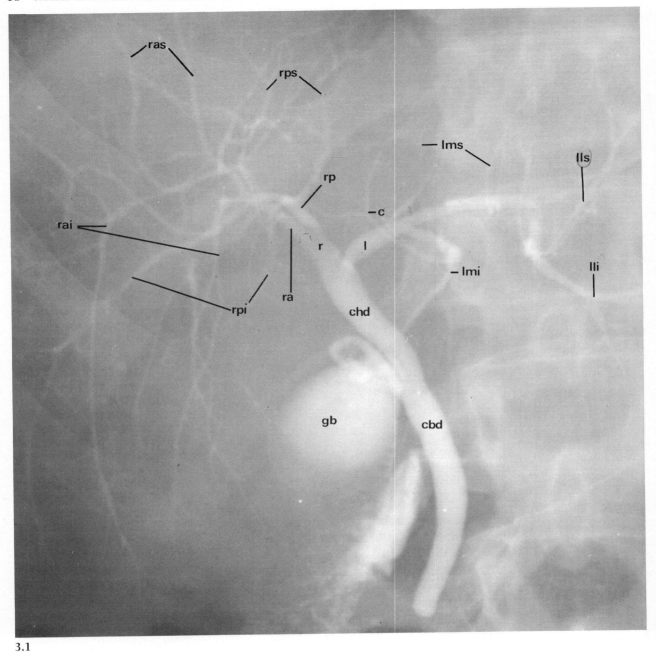

3.1

3.1 Normal intrahepatic duct pattern in the antero-posterior position, shown *at endoscopic cholangiography* (for key to lettering see p. 16)

3.2 Normal intrahepatic duct pattern in right posterior oblique position shown *at endoscopic cholangiography*

3.3 *Normal endoscopic cholangiogram* The right posterior area ducts and the right anterior segment ducts unite almost immediately before joining the left hepatic duct so that the right hepatic duct is very short; the left area ducts are well shown

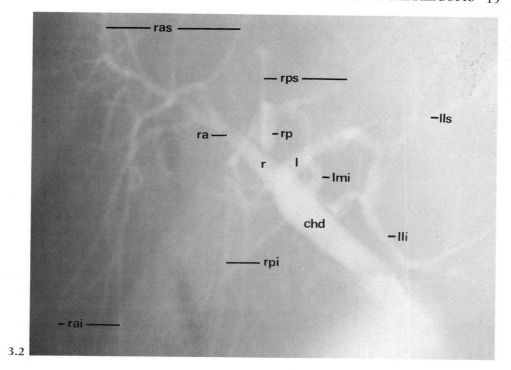

3.2

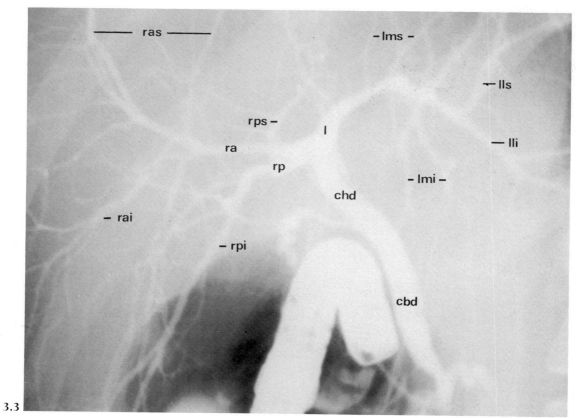

3.3

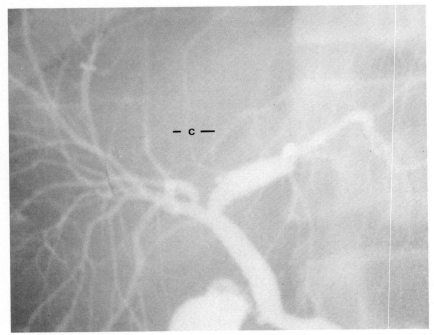

3.4

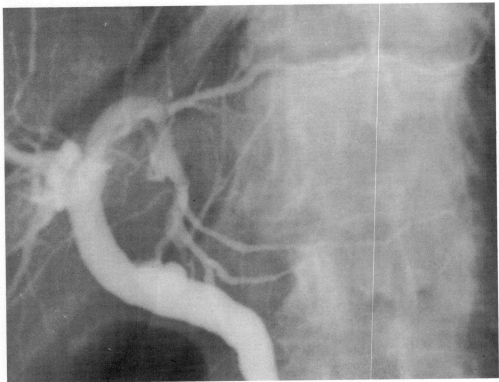

3.5

3.4 Ducts draining the caudate lobe join both right and left hepatic ducts, shown *at endoscopic cholangiography*

3.5 *Endoscopic cholangiogram* Normal ducts in the left lateral segment with marked curvature of the inferior ducts

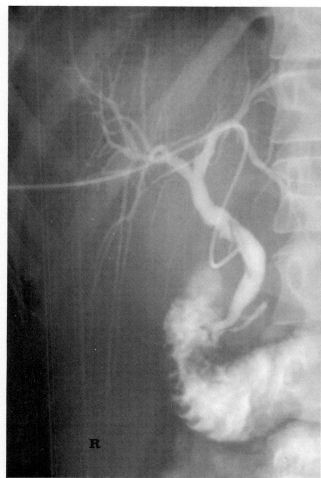

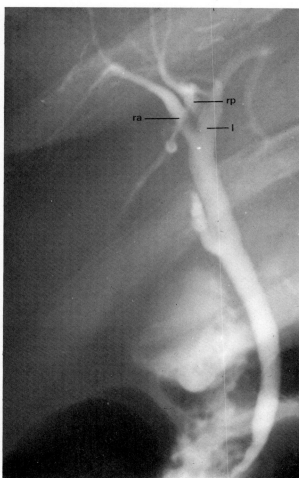

3.6

3.7

3.6 **Riedel's lobe** *T-tube cholangiogram* Right inferior area ducts both anterior and posterior extend downward into Riedel's lobe (R); there is some reflux into the pancreatic duct

3.7 *Endoscopic cholangiogram* The right posterior segment duct drains directly into the left hepatic duct

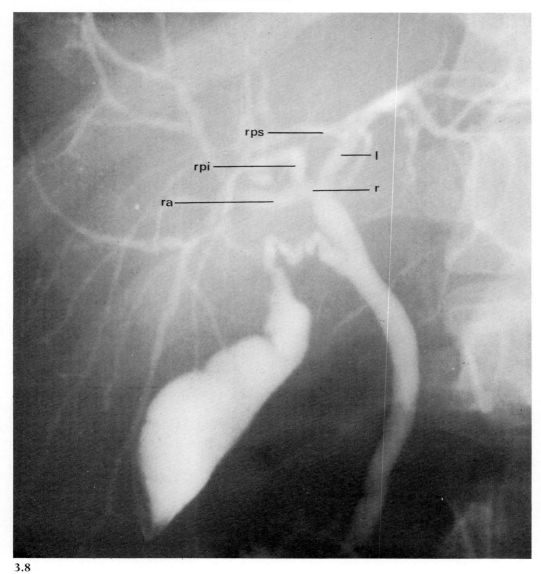

3.8

3.8 *Endoscopic cholangiogram* The right posterior superior area duct drains directly into the left hepatic duct

3.9 *Normal intravenous cholangiogram (90 minutes)* The right and left hepatic ducts are demonstrated. The common hepatic and common bile duct taper towards the papilla. There is good opacification of the gallbladder
3.10 *Normal endoscopic cholangiogram and pancreatogram*

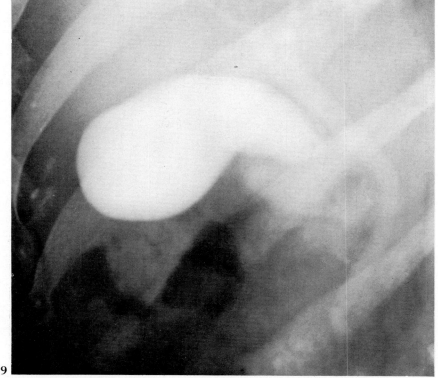

3.9

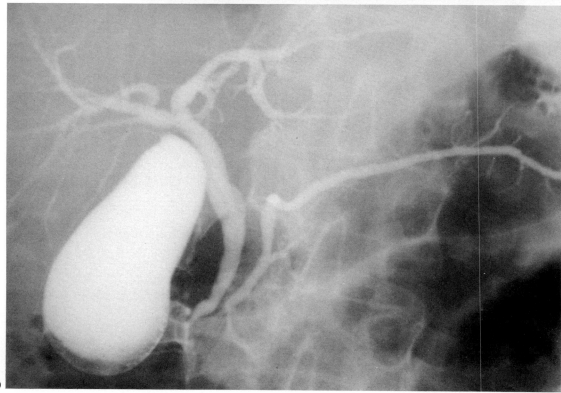

3.10

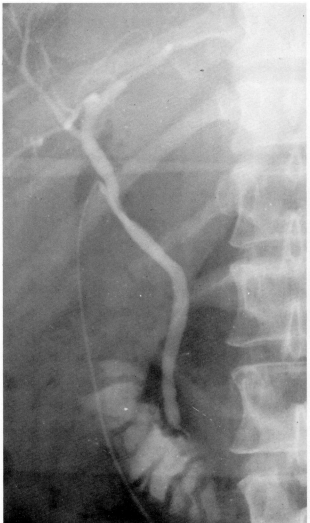

3.11

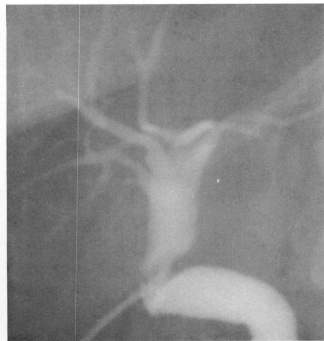

3.12

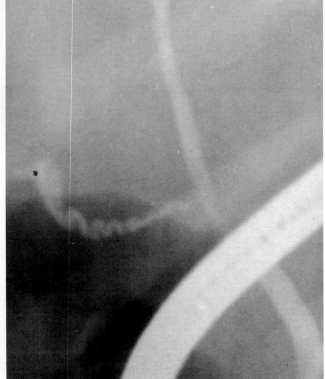

3.13

3.11 *Normal operative cholangiogram after cholecystectomy*
Contrast medium outlines the bile duct and has entered the
duodenum
3.12 *T-tube cholangiogram* Four ducts unite to form the
common hepatic duct
3.13 *Normal endoscopic cholangiogram* The cystic duct is
inserted at right angles into the right side of the common
hepatic duct

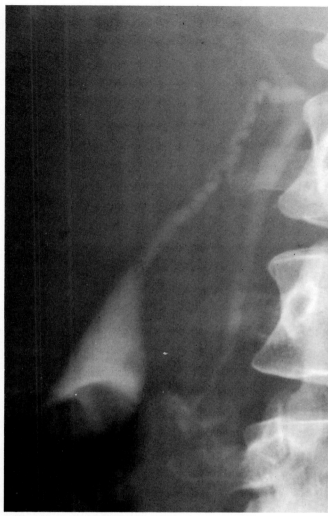

3.14

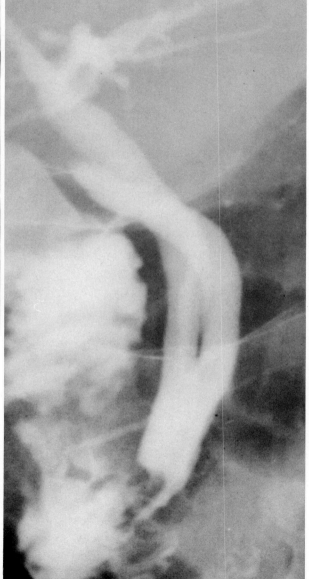

3.15

3.14 **High insertion of cystic duct** *Intravenous
cholangiogram* The cystic duct joins the common duct
high up near the porta hepatis
3.15 **Low insertion of cystic duct** *Endoscopic
cholangiogram* Low insertion of the cystic duct into the
common hepatic duct and a short common bile duct

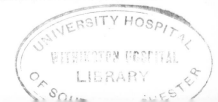

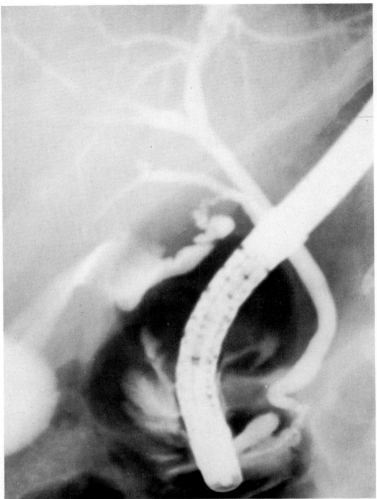

3.16

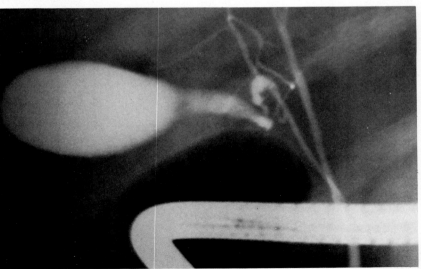

3.17

3.16 **Anomalous extrahepatic duct** *Endoscopic cholangiogram* A right inferior area duct unites with the cystic duct before it joins the common hepatic duct

3.17 **Anomalous extrahepatic duct** *Endoscopic cholangiogram* The right and left hepatic ducts do not unite until they reach the level of the neck of the pancreas. The cystic duct drains into the right hepatic duct

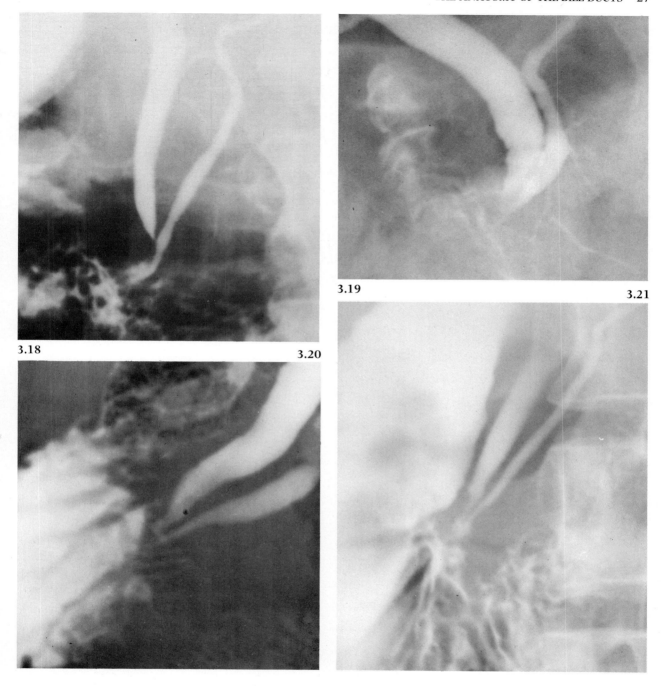

3.18 Long pancreatico-biliary channel *Endoscopic cholangiogram and pancreatogram* The papilla is in the third part of the duodenum

3.19 Short pancreatico-biliary channel *Endoscopic cholangiogram and pancreatogram* View following withdrawal of the endoscope

3.20 *Endoscopic cholangiogram and pancreatogram* There is a common pancreatico-biliary channel

3.21 Ampullary dilatation of the common channel *Endoscopic cholangiogram and pancreatogram* Such dilatation of the channel is seen only occasionally

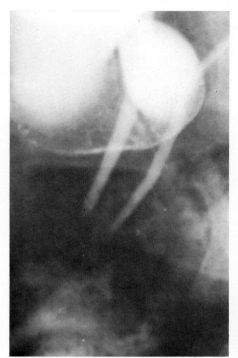

3.22

3.22 **Separate biliary and pancreatic channels** *Endoscopic cholangiogram* Separate orifices for the bile and pancreatic ducts were seen and cannulated endoscopically

3.23 **Pseudo-calculus appearance in lower common bile duct** *Endoscopic cholangiography* A rounded filling defect is sometimes seen at operative or endoscopic cholangiography above the sphincter on the lateral aspect. a *During injection* A rounded filling defect is evident.
(continued on next page)

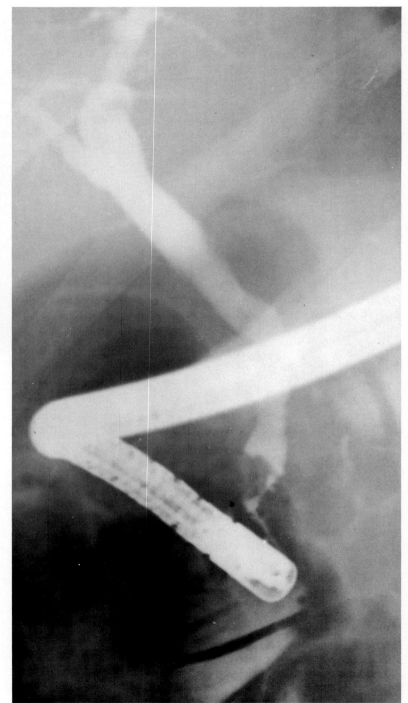

3.23a

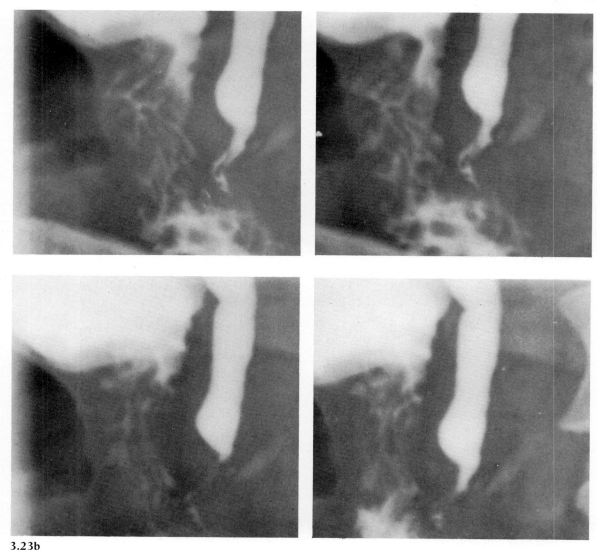

3.23b

b *Serial views several minutes after withdrawal of the endoscope* The sphincter relaxed and the biliary channel has opened up to reveal no evidence of calculi. The pseudocalculus sign is probably due to buckling of the bile duct mucosa above the sphincter of Oddi

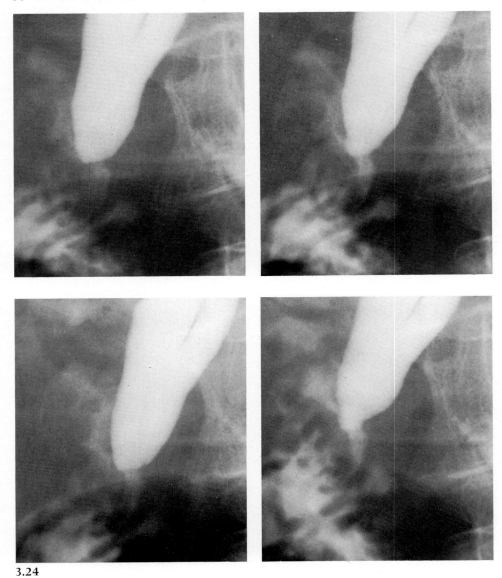

3.24

3.24 Normal distal common bile duct *Fine-needle cholangiogram* The examination was carried out to exclude papillary stenosis. Note the low insertion of the cystic duct

Communicating cavernous ectasia of the intrahepatic ducts (Caroli's disease)

In 1958 Caroli *et al.* described a disease characterized by non-obstructive dilatation of the intrahepatic bile ducts, a marked predisposition to biliary calculous disease and cholangitis without cirrhosis or portal hypertension and in which the dilated saccular ducts contained bile and communicated freely with the biliary tree and each other.

The disorder may be associated with congenital hepatic fibrosis, renal medullary cystic disease (Mall *et al.* 1974) and choledochal cyst (Gots & Zuidema 1970), and is thought to be congenital because of these associations and because it has been observed in the newborn. Polycystic disease of the liver, although an inherited hepatobiliary disorder, differs from Caroli's disease in that the cysts in this condition do not contain bile and do not communicate with the bile ducts. The prognosis is good in polycystic disease unless there is associated disease of the kidneys, which occurs in about half the patients (Melnick 1955). Malignant change may complicate congenital hepatic fibrosis, Caroli's disease or choledochal cyst (Murray-Lyon *et al.* 1972).

A correct diagnosis of Caroli's disease is difficult prior to surgical exploration. Oral cholecystography or intravenous cholangiography may show calculi, and careful cholangiotomography may show dilated intrahepatic ducts. A liver scan may show decreased areas of uptake which indicates space-occupying lesions. Although some cases have been demonstrated by percutaneous cholangiography the diagnosis is usually made by operative cholangiography (Mujahed *et al.* 1971).

Large solitary cysts communicating with the intrahepatic ducts may occur (Eisen *et al.* 1963). Minor degrees of cystic dilatation of the intrahepatic ducts may be demonstrated incidentally at operative and T-tube cholangiography after cholecystectomy, and similar appearances may be evident following iatrogenic rupture of the intrahepatic bile ducts (Goldman *et al.* 1976). Bile cysts may follow prolonged extrahepatic biliary obstruction of all types (Sherlock 1975).

References

Caroli J., Couinaud C., Soupault R., Porcher P. & Eteve J. (1958) *Sem. Hôp. Paris*, **34**, 496

Eisen H.B., Poller S., Maxwell J.W. & Jackson F.C. (1963) *Radiology*, **81**, 276

Goldman S.M., Diamond A. & Salik J.O. (1976) *Radiology*, **118**, 13

Gots R.E. & Zuidema G.D. (1970) *Amer. J. Surg.*, **119**, 726

Mall J.C., Ghahremani G.G. & Boyer J.L. (1974) *Gastroenterology*, **66**, 1029

Melnick P.J. (1955) *Arch Path.*, **59**, 162

Mujahed Z., Glenn F. & Evans J.A. (1971) *Amer. J. Roentgenol.*, **113**, 21

Murray-Lyon I.M., Shilkin K.B., Laws J.W., Illing R.C. & Williams R. (1972) *Quart. J. Med.*, **41**, 477

Sherlock S. (1975) *Diseases of the Liver and Biliary System*. Oxford: Blackwell Scientific Publications

4 Congenital Disorders of the Bile Ducts

Choledochal cyst

Spherical enlargement of part or all of the common bile duct and adjacent portions of the common hepatic duct is a feature of this disease which occurs more commonly in females and often presents before 10 years of age. The cysts are usually single and large, but may be multiple, with a high amylase content (Babbitt 1969). Histologically there is little or no epithelial lining. Abnormally high insertion of the pancreatic duct into the bile duct may play a rôle in the formation of choledochal cyst.

Patients present with intermittent jaundice, pain and abdominal mass or the cyst may perforate (Goswitz & Kimmerling 1966).

A plain X-ray of the abdomen may show a soft tissue mass and barium meal examination may show indentation or anterior bowing of the descending duodenum and displacement of the stomach to the left. Choledochal cysts have been demonstrated by oral cholecystography (Rosenquist 1969) and by intravenous cholangiography (Jones & Olbourne 1973). An ultrasound scan may reveal a transonic space-occupying lesion. Transhepatic cholangiography or operative cholangiography via the gallbladder may be used to outline the cyst.

References

Babbitt D. P. (1969) *Ann. Radiol. (Paris)*, **12**, 231

Goswitz J. T. & Kimmerling R. (1966) *Surgery*, **59**, 878

Jones C. A. & Olbourne N. A. (1973) *Brit. J. Radiol.*, **46**, 711

Rosenquist C. J. (1969) *Brit. J. Radiol.*, **42**, 61

Choledochocoele

Unusual cystic lesions of the terminal common bile duct have been reported under various names, including choledochocoele (Brunton & Bamforth 1972), enterogenous cyst of the ampulla of Vater (Brooks & Weinstein 1943) and intraduodenal choledochal cyst (Serfas & Lyter 1957). The patients have episodic pain and biliary colic, episodes of jaundice and pancreatitis. A well-defined filling defect projecting into the duodenal lumen is seen in the majority at barium meal examination and no filling with barium occurs. Intravenous cholangiography may show club-like dilatation of the terminal common bile duct. The lesion has been shown at duodenoscopy and retrograde cholangiography as well as at operative cholangiography. In the series reported by Schotz et al. (1976), six out of sixteen patients had stones at the time of diagnosis or in the past, while the remainder were never shown to have had biliary calculi.

References

Brooks B. & Weinstein A. (1943) *Ann. Surg.*, **117**, 728

Brunton F. J. & Bamforth J. (1972) *Gut*, **13**, 207

Schotz F. J., Carrera G. F. & Larson C. R. (1976) *Radiology*, **118**, 25

Serfas L. S. & Lyter C. S. (1957) *Amer. J. Surg.*, **93**, 979

Biliary atresia

Atresia of the bile ducts produces jaundice in infants which increases slowly and progressively over a period of weeks. The bile ducts may be entirely absent or replaced by fibrous strands, and the gallbladder may also be absent or the biliary tract represented only by a gallbladder connected directly with the duodenum. About 15 to 29 per cent. of cases present with atresia of the extrahepatic ducts alone which is potentially correctable by surgical by-pass. Operative cholangiography is used to outline the existing duct system (Hays et al. 1967) and at operation patent bile ducts distal to the atresia are found to contain no bile and to be hypoplastic.

Congenital biliary hypoplasia is characterized by recurrent bouts of cholestasis in childhood (Longmire 1964). The extrahepatic bile ducts are narrowed but patent, and hepatic histology may show decreased or absent bile ducts in the portal zone (Haas & Dobbs 1958). The condition may be hereditary and the prognosis is relatively good. Hypoplasia of the biliary tree may also occur in mucoviscidosis.

Congenital bronchobiliary fistula has been described and is extremely rare but has been demonstrated at cholangiography (Enjoji et al. 1963).

References

Enjoji M. Watanabe H. & Nakamura Y. (1963) *Ann. paediat. (Basel)*, **200**, 321

Haas L. & Dobbs R. H. (1958) *Arch. Dis. Childh.*, **33**, 396

Hays D. M., Woolley M. M., Snyder W. H., Reed G. B., Gwinn J. L. & Landing B. H. (1967) *J. Pediat.*, **71**, 598

Longmire W. P. (1964) *Ann. Surg.*, **159**, 335

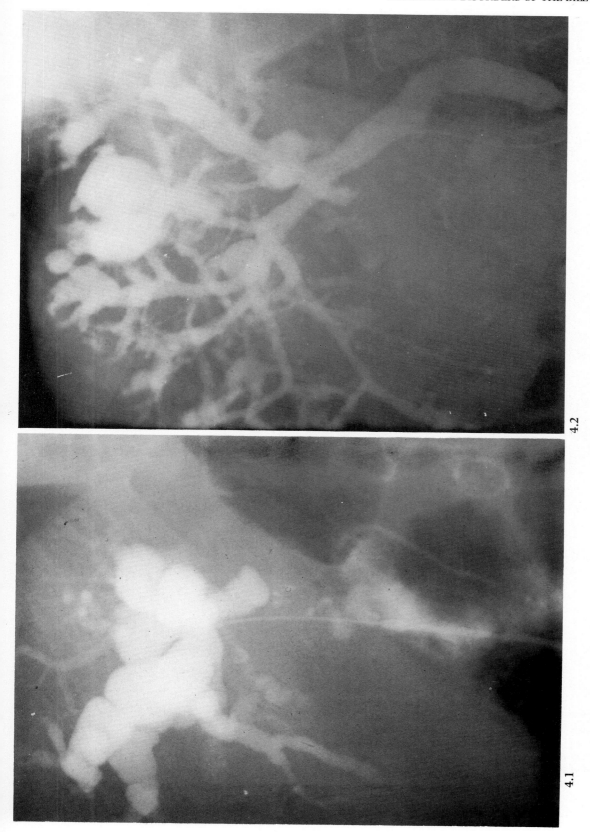

4.1

4.1 **Cavernous ectasia of the intrahepatic bile ducts** *Percutaneous cholangiogram* The intrahepatic ducts in both lobes are dilated, although the common duct is normal in calibre. (Courtesy of Dr. R.D. Dick)

4.2 **Cavernous ectasia of the intrahepatic bile ducts** *Operative cholangiogram* In addition to the dilated intrahepatic ducts there is a calculus in the lower common bile duct. (Courtesy of Prof. G.H. Whitehouse)

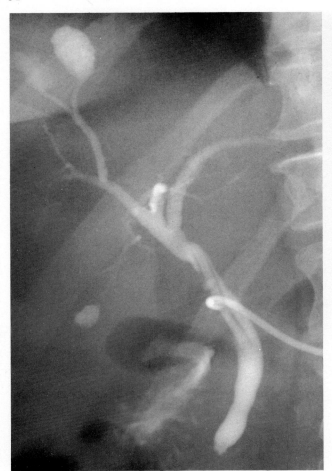

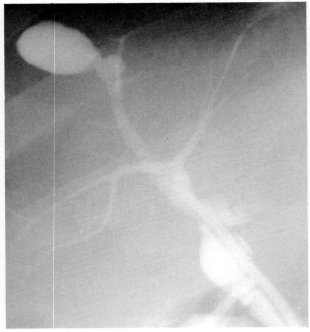

4.4

4.3

4.3 Cystic dilatation of ducts in the right lobe of the liver *T-tube cholangiogram* The duct dilatation shown here was found incidentally in a patient who had undergone cholecystectomy for gallbladder stones. No common-duct stones were present at operation

4.4 Cystic dilatation of intrahepatic and extrahepatic bile ducts *T-tube cholangiogram* The common hepatic duct, the confluence of the right and left hepatic ducts and a branch duct in the right lobe are dilated. The patient had presented with jaundice due to a common bile duct stone. (Courtesy of Dr. E.W.L. Fletcher)

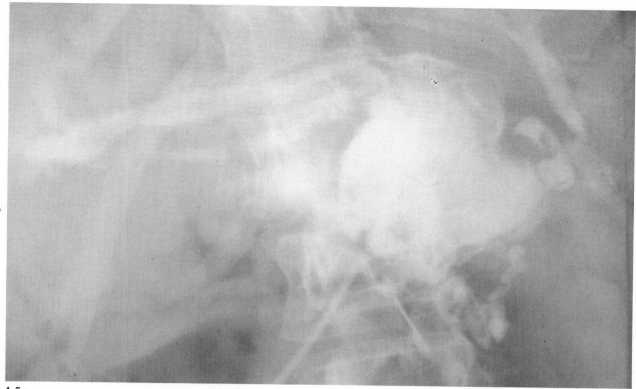

4.5a

4.5b

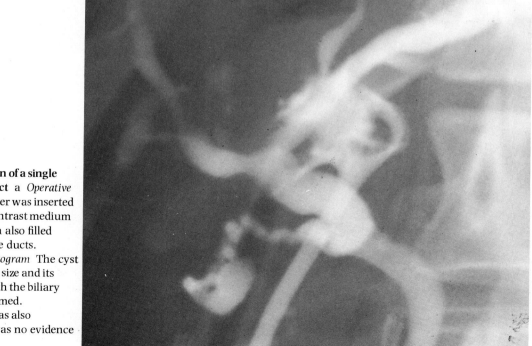

4.5 Cystic dilatation of a single intrahepatic bile duct a *Operative cystogram* A catheter was inserted into the cyst and contrast medium was injected, which also filled the intrahepatic bile ducts.
b *Post-operative cystogram* The cyst has been reduced in size and its communication with the biliary tree has been confirmed. Cholecystectomy was also performed. There was no evidence of hydatid disease

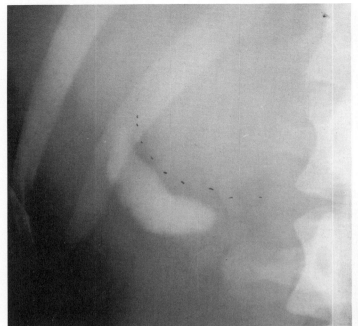

4.6a

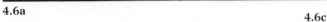

4.6c

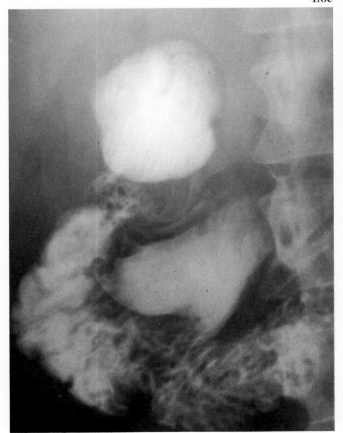

4.6b

4.6 **Choledochal cyst** a *Oral cholecystogram* The gallbladder is displaced around the cyst. b *Intravenous cholangiogram* There is cystic dilatation of the common hepatic duct as well as the common bile duct. c *Barium meal* Film taken after the cyst had been anastomosed directly to the duodenum. (Courtesy of Prof. J.H. Middlemiss)

4.7 **Choledochal cyst** (Jones & Olbourne 1973) a *Intravenous cholangiogram* The common bile duct shows cystic dilatation but the gallbladder is normal in size. b *Tomogram* A radiolucent calculus is shown within the dilated common bile duct

4.8 **Choledochal cyst** a *Endoscopic cholangiogram and pancreatogram* There is cystic dilatation of the intrahepatic bile ducts in addition to the large choledochal cyst. The bile and pancreatic ducts unite two centimeteres proximal to the papilla, and the Santorini and Wirsung ducts in the head are displaced downwards by the cyst. b *Operative cholangiogram* Contrast medium has refluxed retrogradely into the pancreatic duct. (Courtesy of Dr. J.F. Rey)

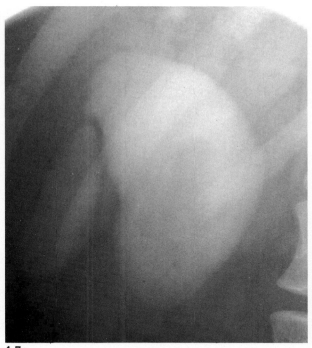

4.7a

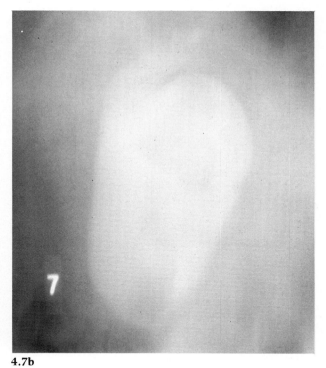

4.7b

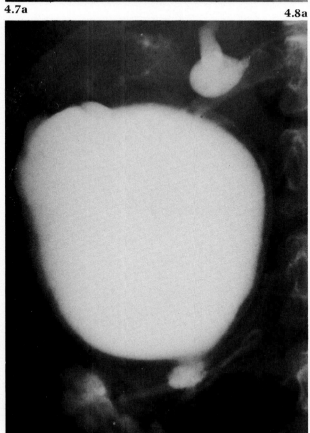

4.8a

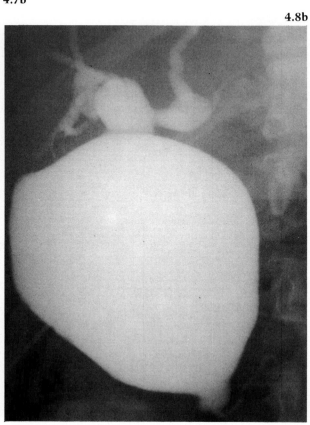

4.8b

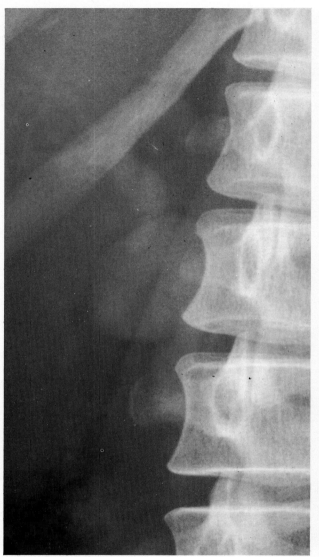

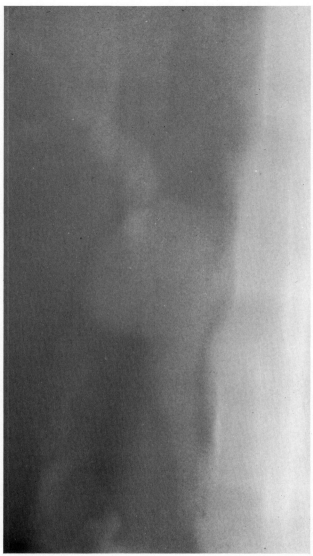

4.9a

4.9b

4.9 Choledochal cyst a *Intravenous cholangiogram* Cystic dilatation of the proximal part of the common bile duct is seen.
b *Tomogram* (Courtesy of Dr. P.B. Galvin)

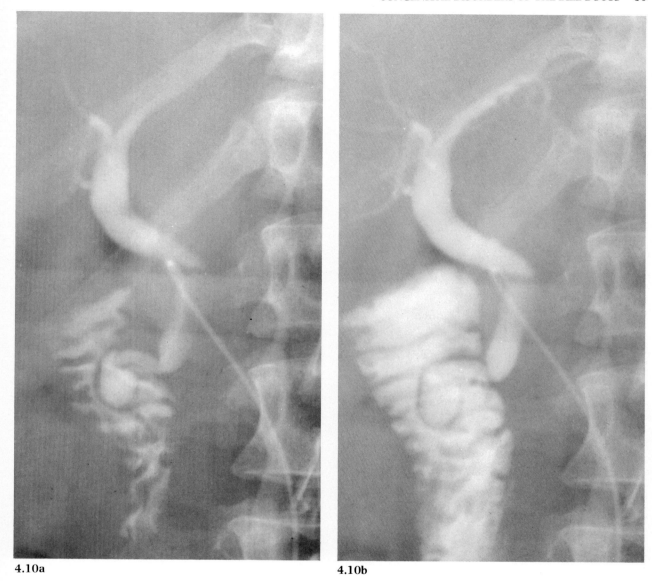

4.10a

4.10b

4.10 **Choledochocoele** a & b *Operative cholangiogram* Films taken during cholecystectomy for gallbladder stones. No bile duct calculi are evident. There is dilatation of the terminal portion of the common bile duct which protrudes into the duodenum, and no hold-up of contrast medium

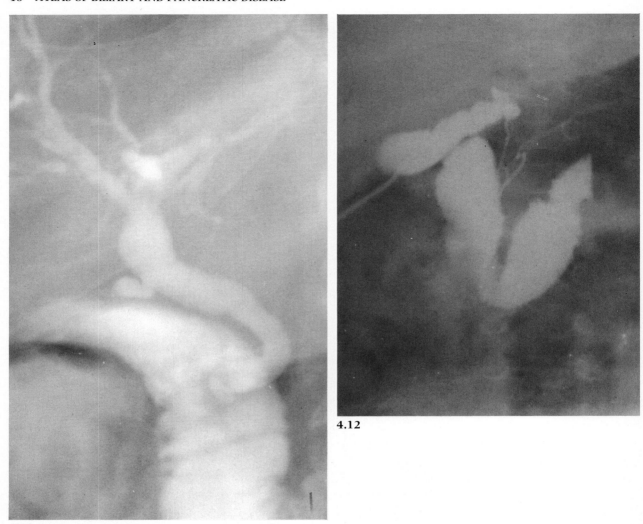

4.11

4.12

4.11 **Choledochocoele** The patient had post cholecystectomy pain. *Endoscopic cholangiogram* The terminal common bile duct is dilated, protrudes into the duodenum and contains a small stone

4.12 **Biliary atresia** *Operative cholangiogram* Contrast medium has not filled the proximal bile ducts because of atresia. The common bile duct is hypoplastic and the pancreatic duct has filled retrogradely

The anatomy of the gallbladder

The gallbladder has a capacity of 30 to 50 ml and lies on the undersurface of the right lobe of the liver in the gallbladder fossa adjacent to the duodenal bulb and above the hepatic flexure of the colon. The fundus of the gallbladder usually lies anteriorly, and its body extends into a narrow neck which continues into the cystic duct. The proximal portion of the duct has a convoluted fold pattern due to the valves of Heister and it is in this region that stones may become impacted. More distally, the cystic duct is usually wider with a smooth mucosal pattern. Dilatation of the neck of the gallbladder, referred to as Hartmann's pouch, is now considered to be the result of pathological processes and is not a normal anatomical finding (Hand 1973). The gallbladder wall consists of three layers: an outer serous layer formed by the peritoneum which covers the major portion of the gallbladder except that part of the body and neck that are in contact with the liver; a middle layer composed of muscular and elastic fibres, and an inner mucosal layer of columnar epithelium having no submucosa and loosely attached to the middle layer, sometimes assuming a delicate folded pattern. Rokitansky–Aschoff sinuses may occur and are projections of the mucosa into the middle layer. The mucosa is continuous with that of the bile ducts.

Hepatic bile is stored and concentrated in the gallbladder which contracts in response to the hormone cholecystokinin, which is released from the upper intestine in response to various stimuli including the presence of fat, and protein. Cholecystokinin produces contraction of the normal gallbladder within one or two minutes of entering the blood stream and empties it within 15 minutes.

Oral cholecystography is the best non-invasive method of demonstrating the gallbladder. Non-opacification may be due to alimentary obstruction, impaired liver function or disease of the gallbladder or cystic duct. Re-absorption of oral contrast medium through the wall of the inflamed gallbladder has been suggested as a cause of non-opacification (Berk & Lasser 1964).

Though the gallbladder may be shown quite well by intravenous cholangiography, layering of denser contrast medium against the gallbladder wall is sometimes confusing and may simulate filling defects within the gallbladder lumen. The gallbladder can also be observed at endoscopic or transhepatic cholangiography but disease localized within the gallbladder is not usually an indication for invasive methods. It may also be identified by ultrasonography (Taylor & McCready 1976).

References

Berk R. N. & Lasser E. C. (1964) *Radiology*, **82**, 296

Hand B. H. (1973) *Clin. Gastroent.*, **2**, 3

Taylor K. J. W. & McCready V. R. (1976) *Brit. J. Radiol.*, **49**, 224

Anomalies of the gallbladder

The gallbladder is subject to anomalies of number, form and position which are summarized in Table 5.1.

5 The Anatomy and Congenital Anomalies of the Gallbladder

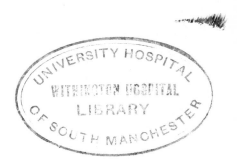

Table 5.1 Congenital anomalies of the gallbladder

Anomalies of primitive foregut bud
    a Failure of bud
       —absent gallbladder and cystic duct
    b Accessory buds or splitting of bud
       —double gallbladder
       —bi-lobed gallbladder
    c Bud migrates to left instead of right
       —left-sided gallbladder

Anomalies of vacuolization of solid gallbladder bud
    —rudimentary gallbladder
    —fundal diverticulum
    —serosal folded gallbladder
    —hourglass gallbladder

Persistent cystohepatic duct
    —diverticulum of body or neck of gallbladder

Persistent intrahepatic gallbladder

Aberrant folding of gallbladder *anlage*
    —retroserosal Phrygian cap

Accessory peritoneal folds
    —floating gallbladder

Congenital absence of the gallbladder and cystic ducts is rare and pre-operative diagnosis may be extremely difficult (Haughton & Lewicki 1973). It may be associated with congenital biliary atresia or anomalous bile ducts but failure to identify the gallbladder at operation is not proof of congenital atresia as it may be intrahepatic or atrophied as a result of cholecystitis. Operative cholangiography is useful in confirming the absence of the gallbladder (Bartone & Grieco 1970).

Double gallbladder is also rare and was found in only three of 9,970 cholecystograms (Boyden 1926). The accessory gallbladder may lie against the normal organ or be situated elsewhere, either in the liver or under its left lobe. The cystic duct may be shared or a second cystic duct may join the common hepatic or an intrahepatic duct. Bi-lobed gallbladder with a longitudinal septum extending from the fundus is also rare with only 10 cases recorded in the literature (Hobby 1970), although a lobulated outline of the fundus is not uncommon.

Transverse septa and strictures of the body of the gallbladder may produce an hourglass deformity evident at oral cholecystography. A similar appearance may be evident in adenomyomatosis, but then filling of Rokitansky–Aschoff sinuses is usually evident on the films taken after a fatty meal. Folding of the body and of the fundus of the gallbladder to produce a 'Phrygian cap' appearance is seen in about 20 per cent. of oral cholecystograms; the folding of the body involves the serosal surface whereas the fundal kinking is usually

retroserosal. Congenital solitary diverticula involving either the body or fundus of the gallbladder may represent remnants – of the embryonic cysto-hepatic ducts or incomplete vacuolization of the gallbladder. Intrahepatic ducts may drain directly into the gallbladder and represent persistent cholecysto-hepatic ducts. Atresia of the common hepatic duct is commonly associated (Jackson & Kelly 1964), and in these circumstances the cystic duct transmits bile directly from the liver to the common bile duct.

The gallbladder may be anomalous in position and lie under the left lobe of the liver, within the liver substance or low down in the right iliac fossa hanging by its own mesentery well below the liver. If the gallbladder does not opacify following oral contrast medium a large film of the whole abdomen including the diaphragm should be taken. A high proportion of patients with intrahepatic gallbladders have gallstones (Bockus 1965).

References

Bartone N. F. & Grieco R. V. (1970) *Amer. J. Roentgenol.*, **110**, 252

Bockus H. E. (1965) *Gastroenterology*, Vol. 3. Philadelphia: Saunders

Boyden E. A. (1926) *Amer. J. Anat.*, **38**, 177

Guyer P. B. & McLoughlin M. (1967) *Brit. J. Radiol.*, **40**, 214

Haughton V. & Lewicki A. W. (1973) *Radiology*, **106**, 305

Hobby J. A. E. (1970) *Brit. J. Surg.*, **57**, 870

Jackson J. B. & Kelly T. R. (1964) *Ann. Surg.*, **159**, 581

Opposite page
5.1 **Normal gallbladder** *Infusion cholangiogram*
5.2 *Endoscopic cholangiogram* The duodenal cap (d) lies between the gallbladder and the common bile duct. The pancreatic duct in the head lies parallel to the bile duct
5.3 **Transverse gallbladder** *Intravenous cholangiogram*

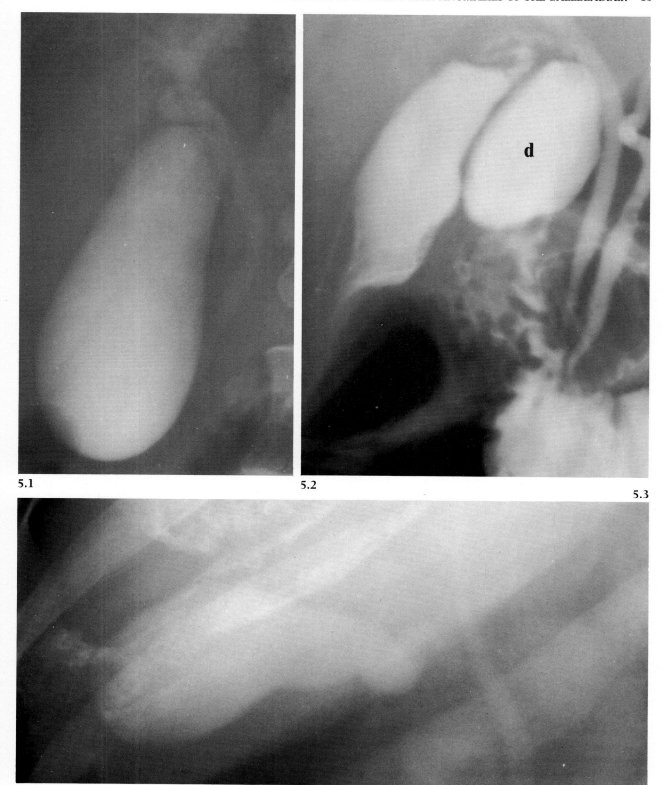

5.1

5.2

5.3

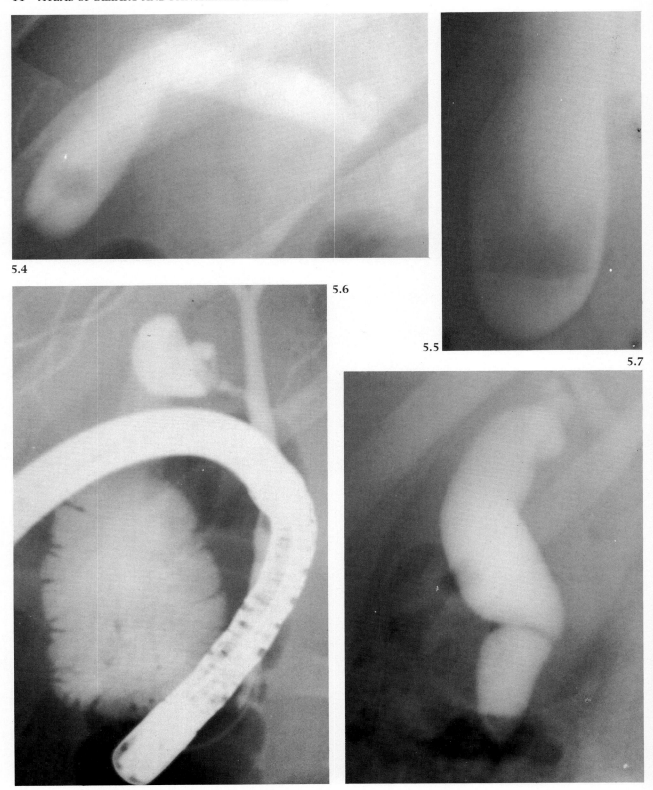

5.4

5.5

5.6

5.7

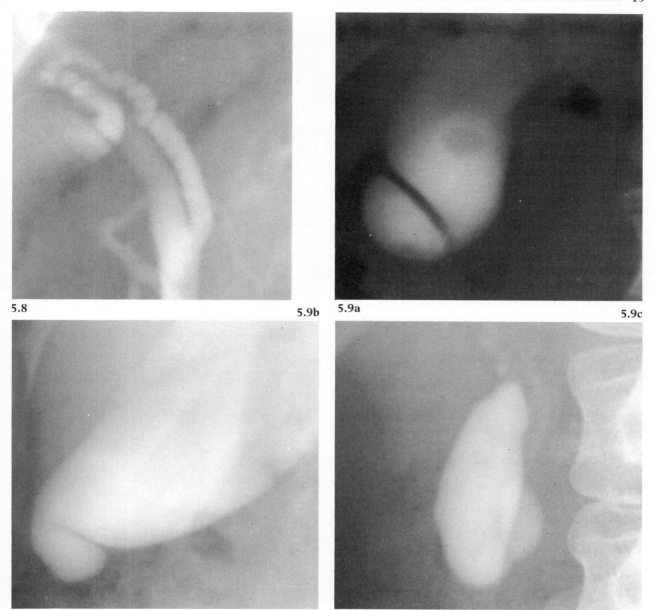

5.8   5.9b   5.9a   5.9c

5.8 *Endoscopic cholangiogram* The cystic duct is convoluted proximally but tends to be smoother and wider as it approaches the bile duct

5.9 a,b,c *Oral cholecystograms* Three examples of retroserosal folding of the fundus of the gallbladder to give the Phyrygian cap deformity. A gallbladder calculus is also present in example a

Opposite page

5.4 **Angled gallbladder** containing a radiolucent calculus. *Oral cholecystogram*

5.5 **Layering of denser contrast medium against the gallbladder mucosa** *Intravenous cholangiogram* Erect film, 90 minutes after injection

5.6 *Normal endoscopic cholangiogram* The mucosa of the normal gallbladder shows a fine linear folded pattern. This is normally obscured by oral or intravenous contrast media

5.7 **Vertical gallbladder** with a transverse fold lying separately from the liver. *Oral cholecystogram*

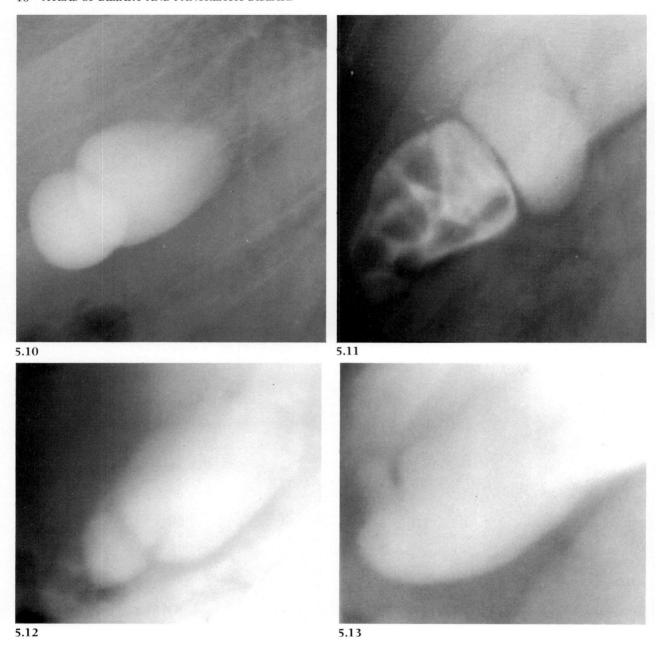

5.10 **Septum of the body of the gallbladder giving an 'hourglass' gallbladder** *Oral cholecystogram*

5.11 **'Hourglass' gallbladder** *Oral cholecystogram* Radiolucent calculi show within the fundal loculus

5.12 **Septa in the body and at the fundus of the gallbladder** *Oral cholecystogram*

5.13 **Congenital diverticulum of the fundus of the gallbladder** *Oral cholecystogram*

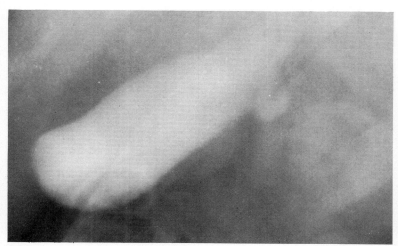

5.14

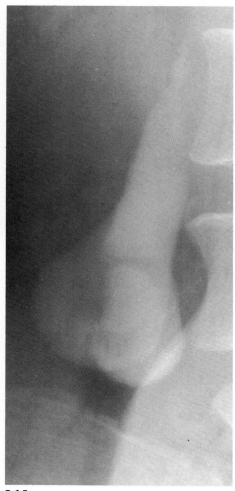

5.15

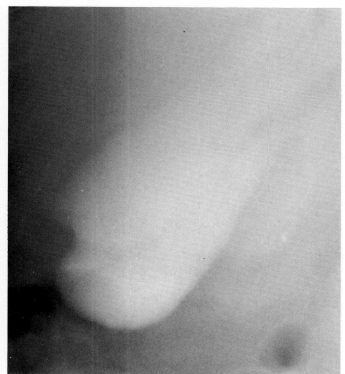

5.16

5.14 **Congenital diverticulum of the neck of the gallbladder** *Oral cholecystogram*
5.15 **Bi-lobed gallbladder** *Oral cholecystogram*
5.16 **Bi-lobed gallbladder** *Oral cholecystogram*

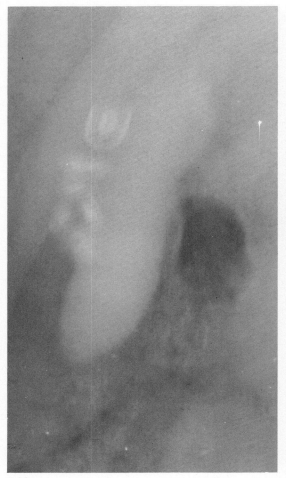

5.17a

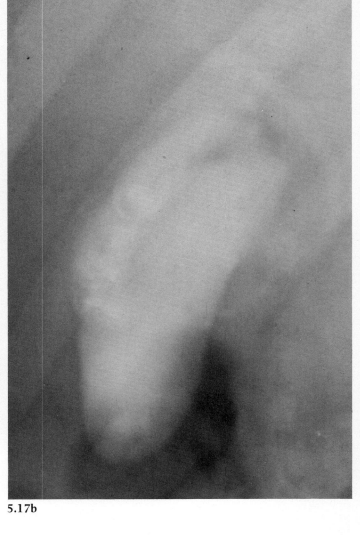

5.17b

5.17 **Double gallbladder** (Guyer & McLoughlin 1967) a *Oral cholecystogram* Opaque calculi are seen lateral to one opacified gallbladder. The second gallbladder which contains the calculi does not function. b *Intravenous cholangiography* has opacified the second gallbladder

Opposite page
5.18 **Intrahepatic gallbladder** a *Intravenous cholangiography with tomography* shows dilated intrahepatic ducts. b A rounded collection of contrast medium within the posterior part of the liver is shown on *another tomographic cut.* c *Endoscopic cholangiography* confirmed the presence of a posteriorly placed intrahepatic gallbladder. d *Lateral view*—the pancreatic duct also filled with contrast medium

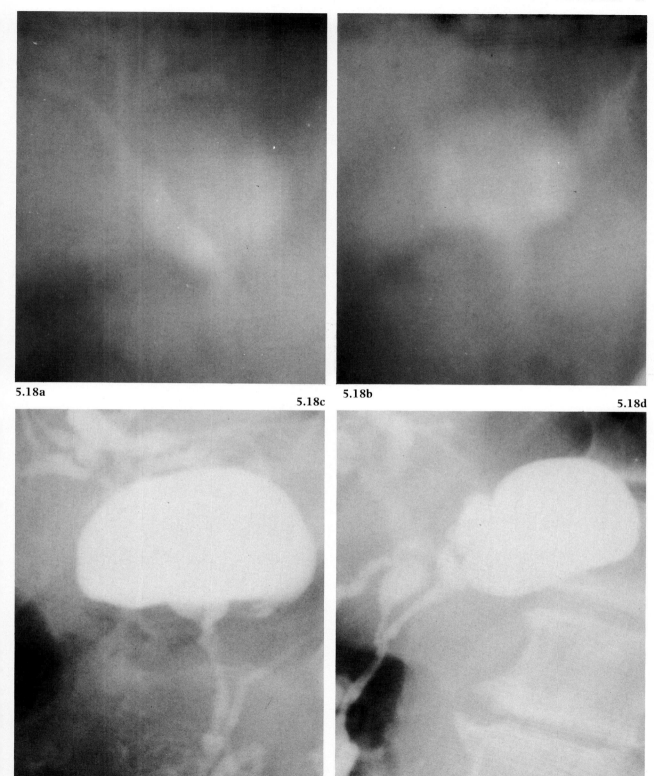

5.18a

5.18c

5.18b

5.18d

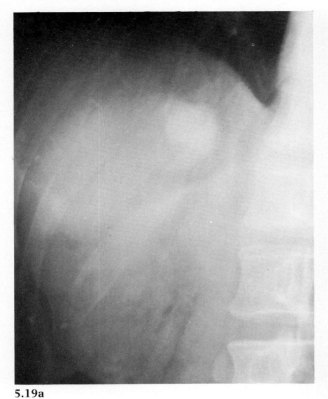

5.19a

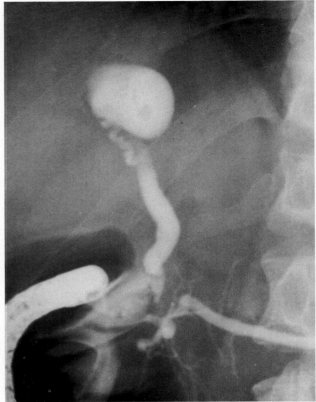

5.19b

5.19 Intrahepatic gallbladder a *Oral cholecystogram* demonstrating the gallbladder within the liver. b *Endoscopic cholangiogram* demonstrating a stone within the intrahepatic gallbladder. The patient has been treated with chenodeoxycholic acid

Cholelithiasis is one of the most common diseases of man and a large number of cholecystectomies and other biliary tract operations are carried out each year for the treatment of biliary tract calculi and their complications.

All gallstones are essentially built up in the same way with pigment at the centre and the remainder of the stone consisting of cholesterol monohydrate, pigment and inorganic calcium salts in different proportions with varying distribution from stone to stone (Bogren 1960). The majority of gallbladder calculi are multiple and of the mixed variety; those composed mainly of pigment are usually multiple and small. Multiple calculi may be faceted due to pressure from adjacent calculi. Pure cholesterol gallstones are less common and are often single and large. About 15 per cent. of gallstones are radiopaque due to the presence of calcium salts which often form a ring round a radiolucent centre, and in some cases the calcium is deposited in layers resulting in a laminated appearance.

Radiopaque gallstones should be differentiated from calcified costal cartilage, renal calculi, and calcified mesenteric lymph glands. Calculi that may look similar to radiopaque gallstones are sometimes found in the appendix. Gas-containing gallstones are rare; the gas is shown radiographically as sharply defined radiolucent crevices in the calculus.

At oral and intravenous cholangiography, gallbladder calculi show as radiolucent filling defects but in a few cases they are of the same or greater density than the contrast medium. In the erect position gallstones may form a horizontal layer in the radiopaque bile.

In the past five years it has been shown that it is possible to dissolve cholesterol-rich gallstones with oral chenodeoxycholic acid (Bell *et al.* 1972; Thistle & Hofmann 1973) and it is important to predict which gallstones are most likely to respond to this type of medical treatment. It has been shown that although radiology is sometimes misleading when the stones are small and irregular, large radiolucent stones with a smooth profile are invariably cholesterol-rich (Bell *et al.* 1975).

Calculi are present in the bile ducts (choledocholithiasis) either secondary to migration from the gallbladder or less commonly as a result of being formed primarily in the bile ducts. Primary duct calculi usually result from stasis due to such conditions as bile duct strictures, stenosis of the papilla of Vater or an impacted calculus. Most of the primary calculi in the common bile duct are single and are usually present in ducts that are dilated whereas secondary duct calculi are usually multiple (Madden 1973). Primary intrahepatic duct calculi are common in South-east Asia where they occur in patients with recurrent pyogenic cholangitis (Wen & Lee 1972; Wastie & Cunningham 1973). Calculi present in the bile ducts of patients who have had a previous cholecystectomy are either primary calculi due to stasis or secondary ones that have been overlooked at operation.

The usual clinical presenting feature of bile duct calculi is colicky right upper quadrant abdominal pain, which may be associated with jaundice and sometimes with fever. Pancreatitis due to calculi passing through or becoming impacted in the ampulla of Vater is another mode of presentation.

Patients being investigated for suspected bile duct calculi should have a plain X-ray film of the abdomen before proceeding to contrast

6 Cholelithiasis

examinations. Infusion cholangiography with tomography is the examination of choice for demonstrating bile duct calculi and should be the initial contrast investigation when liver function is normal.

The development of retrograde cholangiography has added a new dimension to the search for bile duct calculi in patients with abnormal liver function. In some cases it is possible to remove calculi from the duct by performing endoscopic sphincterotomy which allows residual calculi to pass into the duodenum.

Percutaneous cholangiography is useful for demonstrating bile duct calculi if there is failure to cannulate the duct at retrograde cholangiography or when further information about the proximal ducts is required because of total obstruction demonstrated at retrograde cholangiography. Percutaneous cholangiography using the small-bore Chiba needle has proved very useful in the investigation of patients with cholestasis (Elias *et al.* 1975).

Operative cholangiography should always be carried out in patients undergoing biliary tract surgery to reduce the chances of leaving residual calculi in the ducts. Where a T-tube is left to drain the bile ducts, cholangiography should be carried out before it is removed. This is one of the best methods available for demonstrating the bile ducts and establishing finally whether any residual calculi remain in the intrahepatic or extrahepatic ducts, and for establishing that the ampulla of Vater is patent. The T-tube can be used in a therapeutic manner where residual calculi are present in the ducts. The infusion of a bile salt (sodium cholate) solution through the T-tube dissolved about half the residual calculi in one group of patients (Way *et al.* 1972). Residual calculi can also be removed from the duct using a Desjardins forceps or a Dormia ureteral basket introduced through the T-tube track (Magarey 1971; Way *et al.* 1972; Burhenne 1973).

References

Bell G. D., Dowling R. H., Whitney B. & Sutor D. J. (1975) *Gut*, **16**, 359

Bell G. D., Whitney B. & Dowling R. H. (1972) *Lancet*, **ii**, 1213

Bogren H. (1964) *Acta Radiol. Suppl.*, **226**, 37

Bryan G. (1971) *X-Ray Focus*, **11**, 15

Burhenne H. J. (1973) *Amer. J. Roentgenol.*, **117**, 388

Burwood R. J., Davies G. T., Lawrie B. W., Blumgart L. H. & Salmon P. R. (1973) *Clin. Radiol.*, **24**, 397

Elias E., Hamlyn A. N., Jain S., Long R., Summerfield J. A., Dick R. & Sherlock S. (1975) *Gut*, **16**, 831

Madden J. L. (1973) *Surg. Clin. N. Amer.*, **53**, 1095

Magarey C. J. (1971) *Lancet*, **i**, 1044

Nolan D. J. & Gibson M. J. (1970) *Brit. J. Radiol.*, **43**, 652

Thistle J. L. & Hofmann A. F. (1973) *New Engl. J. Med.*, **289**, 655

Wastie M. L. & Cunningham I. G. E. (1973) *Amer. J. Roentgenol.*, **119**, 71

Way L. W., Admirand W. H. & Dunphy J. E. (1972) *Ann. Surg.*, **176**, 347

Wen C. C. & Lee H. C. (1972) *Ann. Surg.*, **175**, 166

Wright F. W. (1977) *Clin Radiol.*, **28**, 469

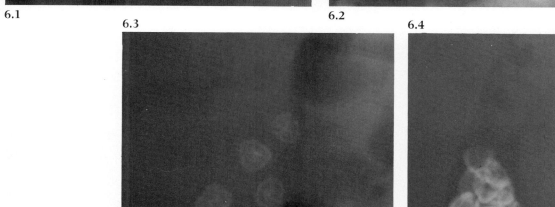

6.1 **Multiple faceted radiopaque gallbladder calculi** *Plain film* One is lodged in Hartmann's pouch

6.2–6.7 **Cholelithiasis** *Plain films* Multiple radiopaque gallbladder calculi of various sizes and shapes

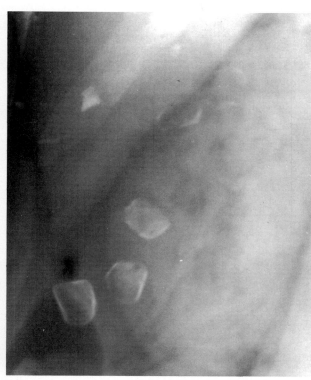

6.1

6.3

6.2

6.4

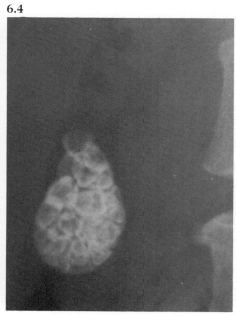

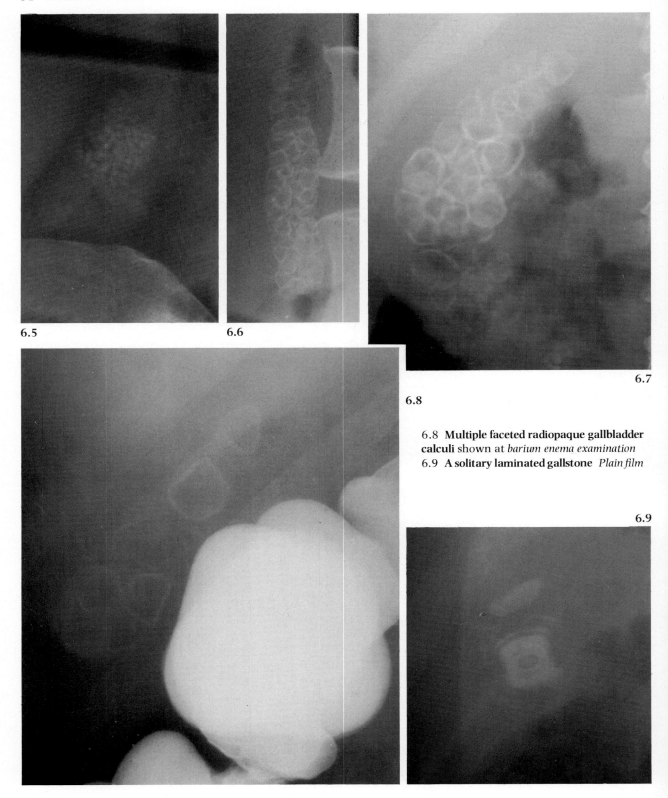

6.5

6.6

6.7

6.8

6.8 **Multiple faceted radiopaque gallbladder calculi** shown at *barium enema examination*
6.9 **A solitary laminated gallstone** *Plain film*

6.9

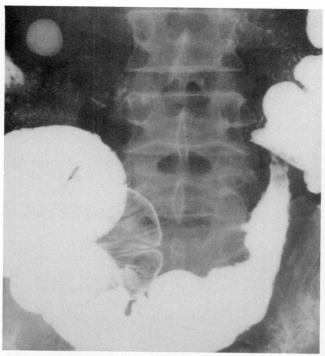

6.10 **Laminated gallstone and Crohn's disease** *Small bowel examination* There is recurrence of Crohn's disease of the ileum, proximal to the site of an ileo-transverse anastomosis. Resection of the terminal ileum and a right hemicolectomy had previously been carried out. Crohn's disease is frequently associated with gallstone formation

6.10

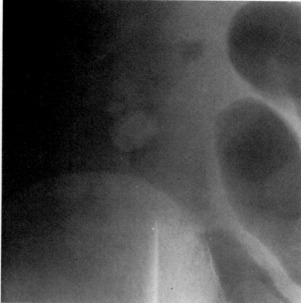

6.11b

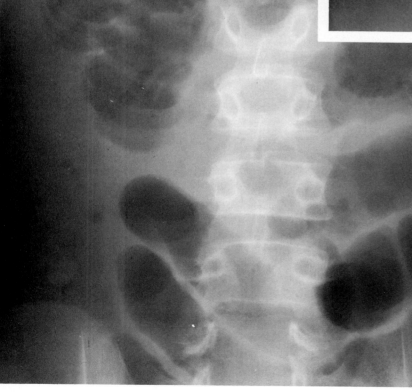

6.11a

6.11 **Appendix calculi** *Plain film* a In this case operation revealed a perforated appendix. There is a high incidence of complications of appendicitis in patients with appendix calculi and immediate appendicectomy is indicated when they are discovered on abdominal radiographs. It is very important to distinguish appendix calculi from gallstones. b enlarged detail

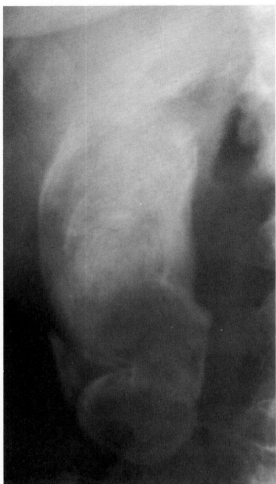

6.12   **6.13**

6.12 **A giant gallbladder calculus** *Plain film* (Courtesy of Dr. J.G. Kenny)

6.13 **Gas-containing gallstones** (Wright 1977) *Plain film* A sharply defined collection of gas is seen in a gallstone

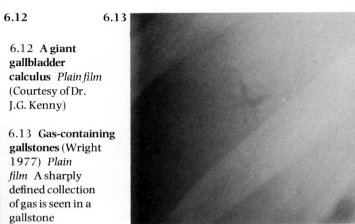

6.14b

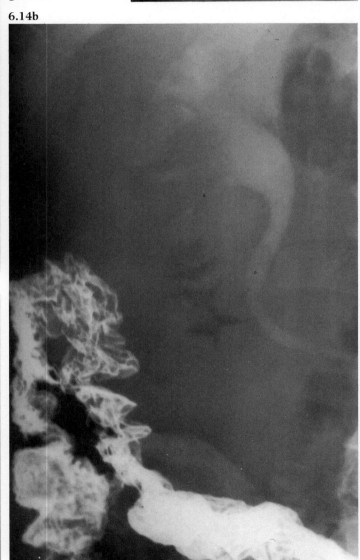

6.14a

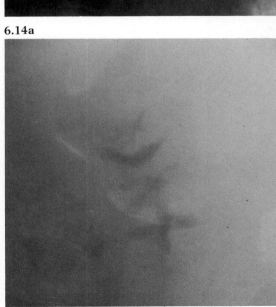

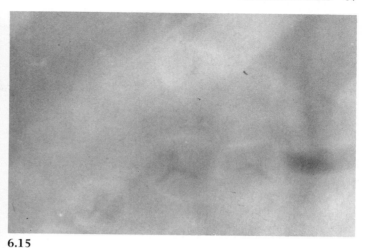

6.15

6.15 **Multiple gas-containing gallstones** *Plain film* The gas patterns are in the shape of the Mercedes-Benz emblem

Opposite page
6.14 **Gas-containing gallstone** (Wright 1977) a *Plain film* Sharply outlined collections of gas with adjacent calcification are shown in the gallbladder area. b *Combined excretion urography and barium meal* The collections of gas are separate from the kidney and colon. c *Radiograph of the excised specimen* Two large calculi are present in the gallbladder. The shape of the calculi suggest that they may have been produced by fracture of a single large stone. The collections of gas are present in one of the calculi

6.16–6.18 **Multiple gallbladder calculi** *Oral cholecystography*

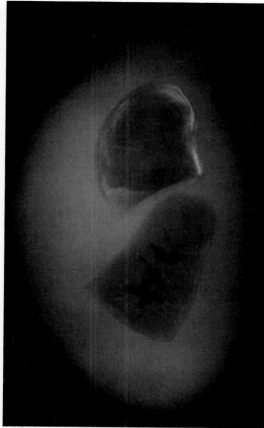

6.14c

6.16 6.17

6.18

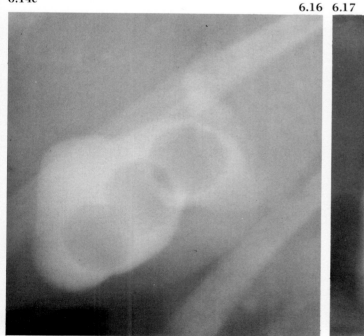

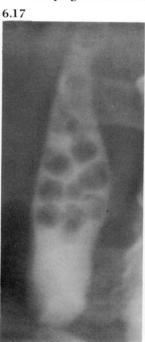

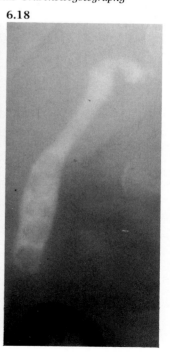

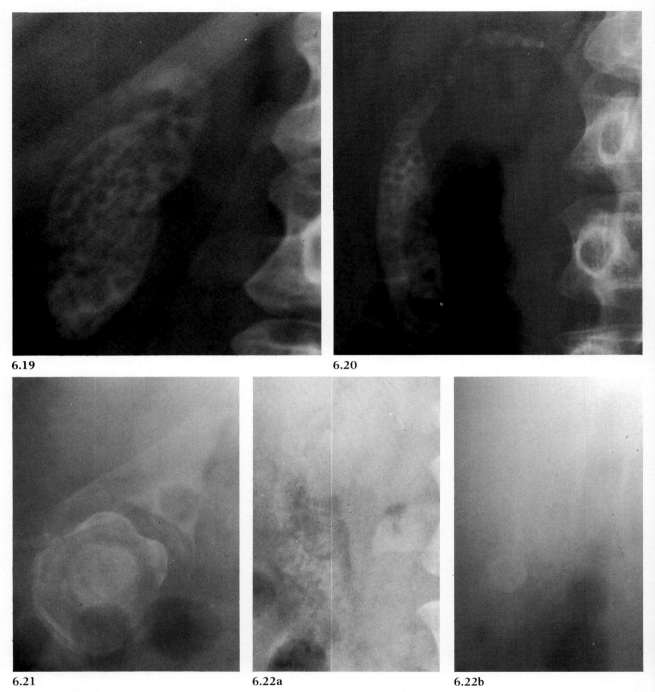

6.19

6.20

6.21

6.22a

6.22b

6.19 **Calculi completely filling the gallbladder** *Oral cholecystogram*

6.20 **Multiple gallbladder calculi** *Oral cholecystogram—after-fat film*

6.21 **Gallbladder calculi** *Oral cholecystogram* There is a large laminated calculus and a smaller radiolucent one present in the gallbladder

6.22 **Gallbladder calculi** *Oral cholecystogram with tomography* a There is very faint visualization of the gallbladder. b Multiple gallbladder calculi are shown on a tomographic cut

6.23 **Solitary gallbladder calculus** *Oral cholecystogram*

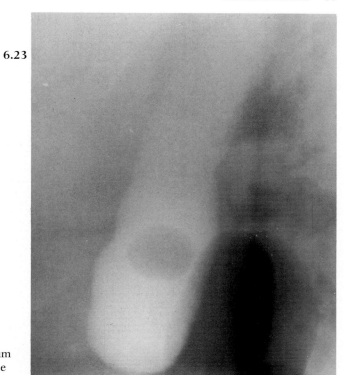

6.23

6.24 **Single small opaque calculus** a *Plain film.* b *Oral cholecystogram* The calculus is obscured by contrast medium in the gallbladder. This example emphasizes the importance of the preliminary plain film

6.24a

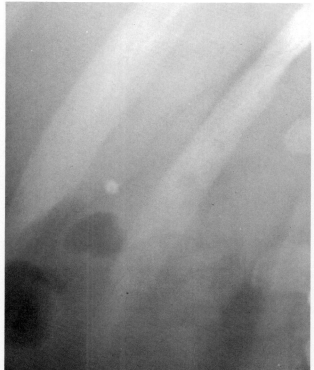

6.24b

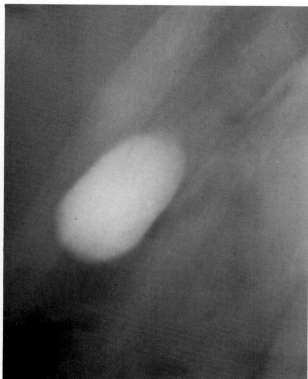

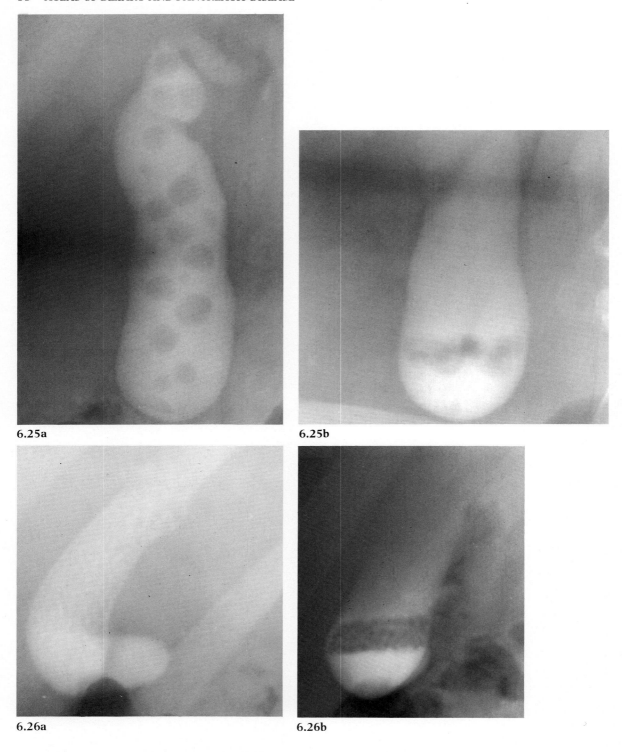

6.25a

6.25b

6.26a

6.26b

6.25, 6.26 **Layering of gallbladder calculi** *Oral cholecystograms* a Radiographs taken prone show calculi dispersed throughout the gallbladder. b Views taken in the erect position show the calculi forming layers

6.27 **Cholelithiasis** (Nolan & Gibson 1970)
Infusion cholangiogram Multiple small calculi are
present in the gallbladder. The bile ducts are
normal. The patient presented following an
episode of biliary colic and jaundice

6.28 **Choledocholithiasis** *Oral cholecystogram
with tomography* The gallbladder failed to
opacify with contrast medium but the bile ducts
opacified and tomography shows two large
calculi in the common bile duct (Courtesy of Dr.
J.G. McNulty)

6.29 **Choledocholithiasis** *Oral cholecystogram
with tomography* Tomography shows bile duct
calculi outlined with contrast medium and that
the gallbladder has not filled (Courtesy of Dr. J.G.
McNulty)

6.27

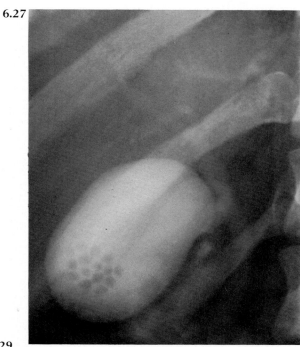

6.28

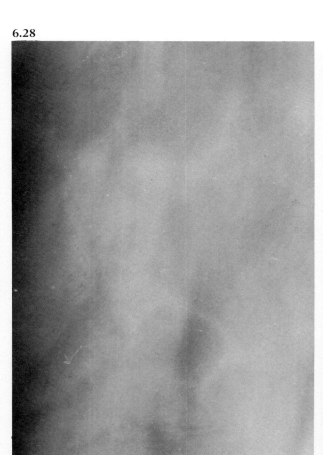

6.29

6.30

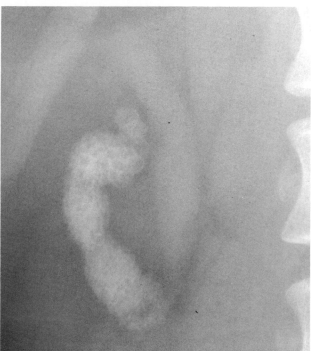

6.30 **Cholelithiasis and cystic duct occlusion** *Oral cholecystogram* Contrast medium outlines the bile ducts but not the gallbladder which is filled with multiple radiopaque calculi. No calculi are present in the bile ducts

6.31 **Cholelithiasis** *Infusion cholangiogram* a The bile ducts are outlined with contrast medium. The distal common bile duct is obscured by overlying gas shadows and no filling defects are evident. b Tomography shows a calculus in the common bile duct and multiple gallbladder calculi. This shows the importance of carrying out tomography to demonstrate the bile ducts adequately at infusion cholangiography

6.31a   6.31b

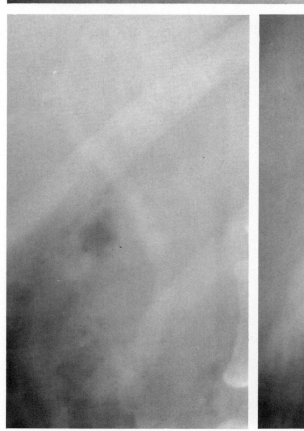

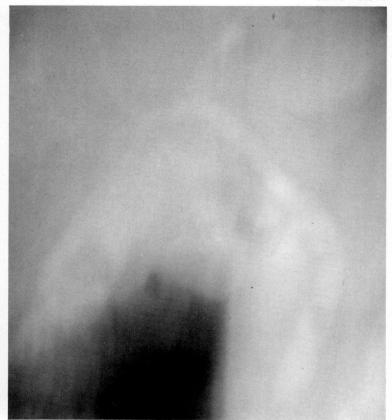

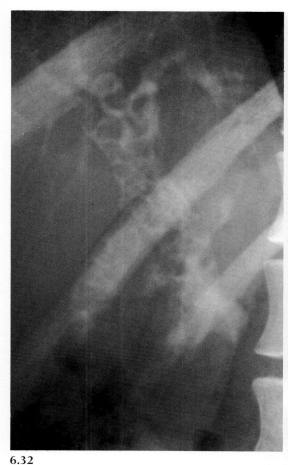

6.32

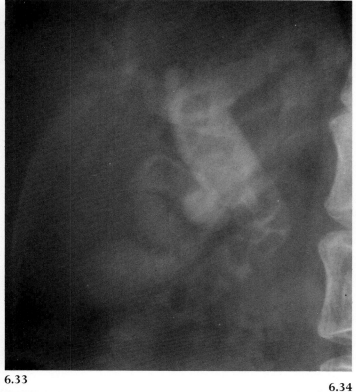

6.33

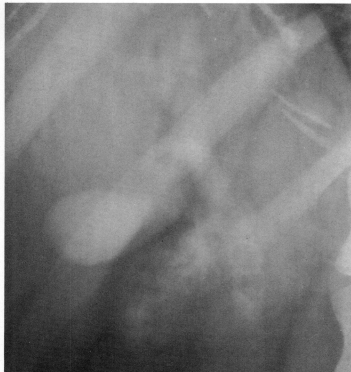

6.34

6.32 **Cholelithiasis** *Infusion cholangiogram* The gallbladder and bile ducts of this 25-year-old female are completely filled with calculi

6.33 **Cholelithiasis** *Infusion cholangiogram* There are a large number of calculi filling the bile and cystic ducts. The gallbladder is contracted and contains a single large calculus

6.34 **Choledocholithiasis** *Infusion cholangiogram* No filling defects are seen in the gallbladder but two calculi are present in the common bile duct. Infusion cholangiography should be carried out to demonstrate the bile ducts in the investigation of biliary colic or an episode of jaundice

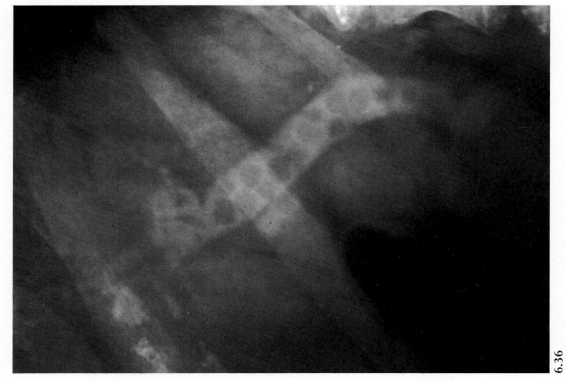

6.36

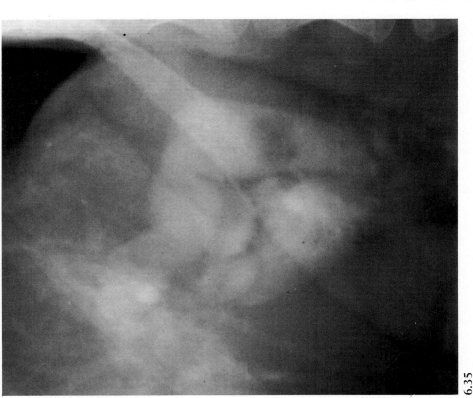

6.35

6.35 **Bile duct calculus** *Infusion cholangiogram* This patient had had a cholecystectomy ten years previously and an infusion cholangiogram was carried out because of abdominal pain and jaundice which had resolved. A solitary calculus is seen in the common bile duct

6.36 **Choledocholithiasis and cystic duct occlusion** (Bryan 1971) *Infusion cholangiogram* A large number of calculi are present in the extrahepatic bile ducts. The gallbladder did not opacify

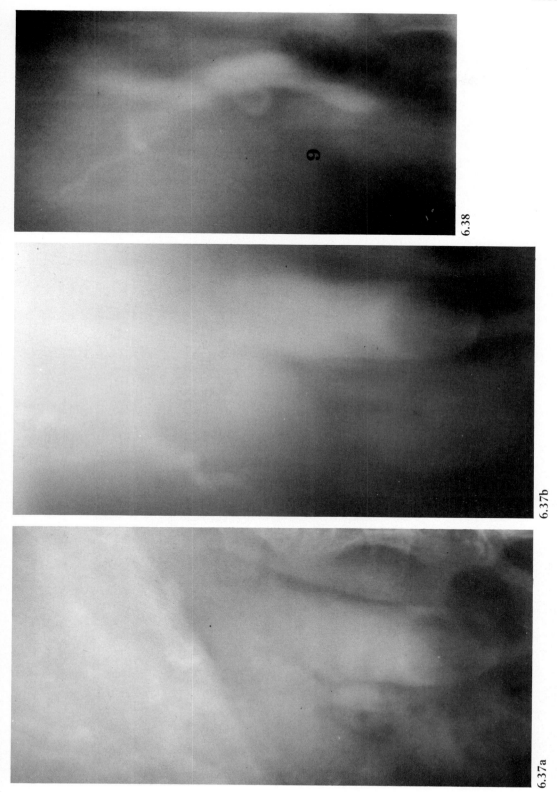

6.38

6.37b

6.37a

6.37 **Bile duct calculus** a *Infusion cholangiogram*   b *With tomogram* A large calculus is shown at the distal end of the common bile duct and the bile ducts are dilated
6.38 **Cystic duct calculus** *Infusion cholangiogram with tomogram at 9cm* A stone is shown occluding the cystic duct

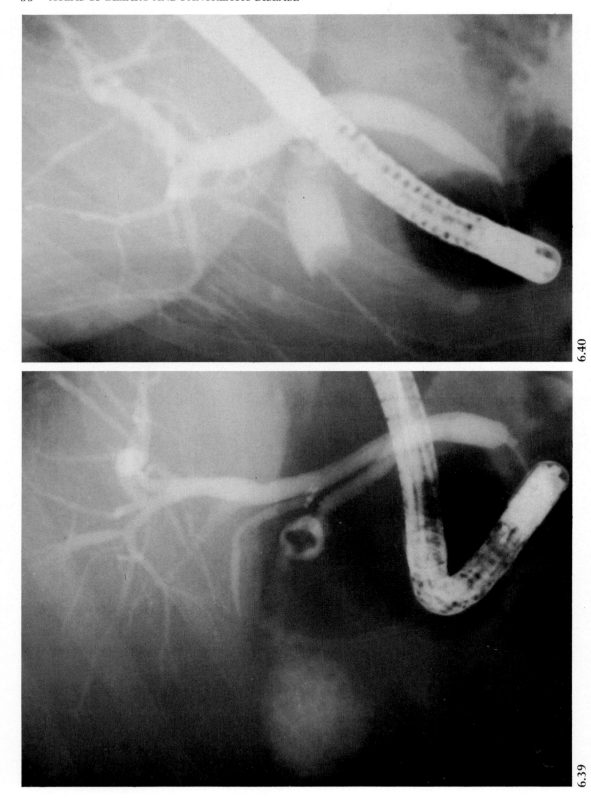

6.39

6.40

6.39 **Cystic duct and gallbladder calculi** (Burwood *et al.* 1973) *Retrograde cholangiogram* Multiple small calculi fill the gallbladder. There are also two calculi, one large and one small in the proximal cystic duct

6.40 **Gallstone impacted in the neck of the gallbladder** *Retrograde cholangiogram* There is indentation of contrast medium in the neck of an unfilled gallbladder

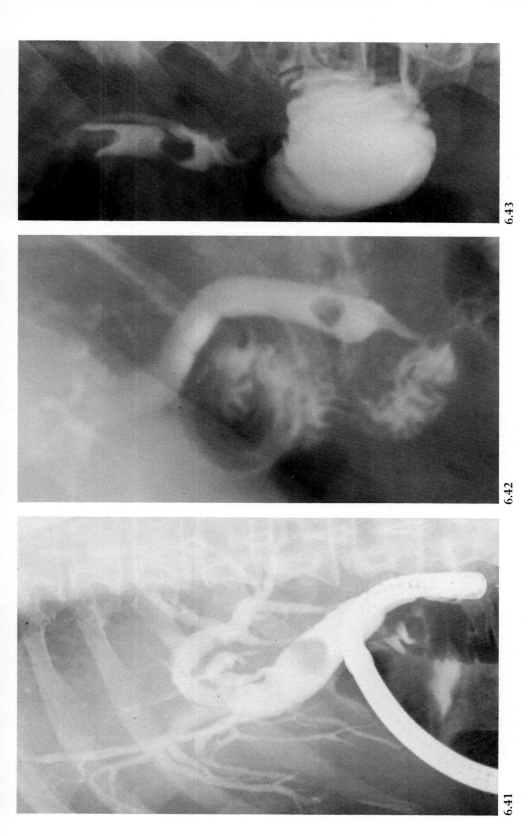

6.41

6.42

6.43

6.41 **Choledocholithiasis** (previous cholecystectomy) *Retrograde cholangiogram* The bile ducts are dilated and a large calculus is present at the junction of the common hepatic and common bile ducts; a small one may also be seen in the left hepatic duct
6.42 **Bile duct calculus** (previous cholecystectomy) *Retrograde cholangiogram* There is a calculus in the common bile duct
6.43 **Choledocholithiasis** *Retrograde cholangiogram* There are multiple calculi in the common bile duct and one of them is causing almost complete obstruction to the retrograde flow of contrast medium

6.44 Bile duct calculus (previous cholecystectomy)
Retrograde cholangiogram A 'Dormia basket' was introduced
through the endoscope in an attempt to remove a residual
calculus from the common bile duct. In this case the
manoeuvre was unsuccessful

6.45 Choledocholithiasis *Retrograde cholangiography and
endoscopic papillotomy* a Two calculi are shown in the distal
end of the common bile duct. An endoscopic papillotomy was
carried out. b One week later a repeat examination shows
that the bile duct calculi are no longer present

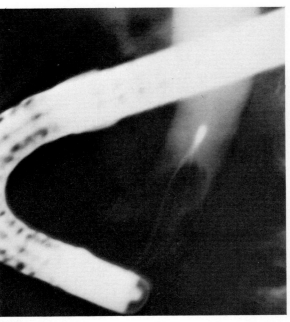

6.45a

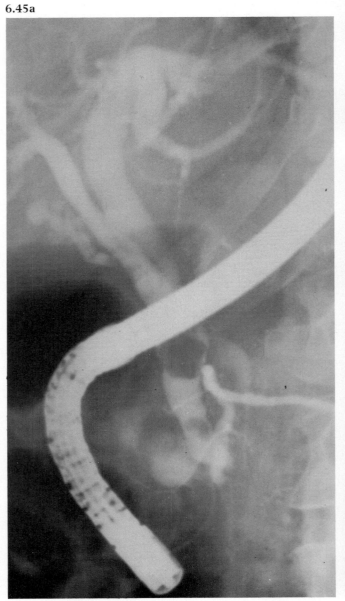

6.44

6.45b

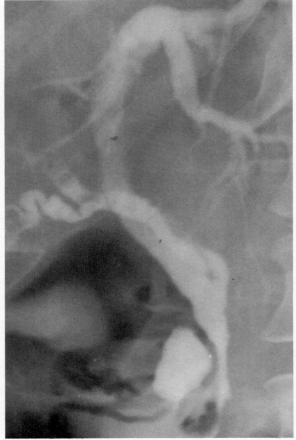

6.46 **Hepatic duct calculus** (previous cholecystectomy) *Percutaneous cholangiogram* There is a very large oval-shaped calculus (8 × 3·5 cm) in the common hepatic duct resulting in marked dilatation of the intrahepatic bile ducts. This is a good example of a primary or stasis-type duct calculus

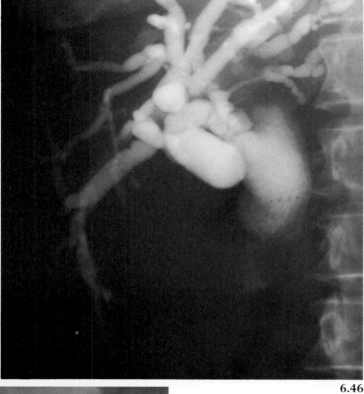

6.46

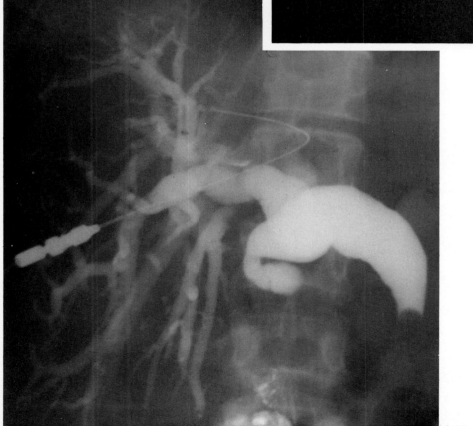

6.47

6.47 **Bile duct calculus** (previous cholecystectomy) *Percutaneous cholangiogram* A calculus is seen obstructing the distal common bile duct, resulting in marked dilatation of the bile ducts

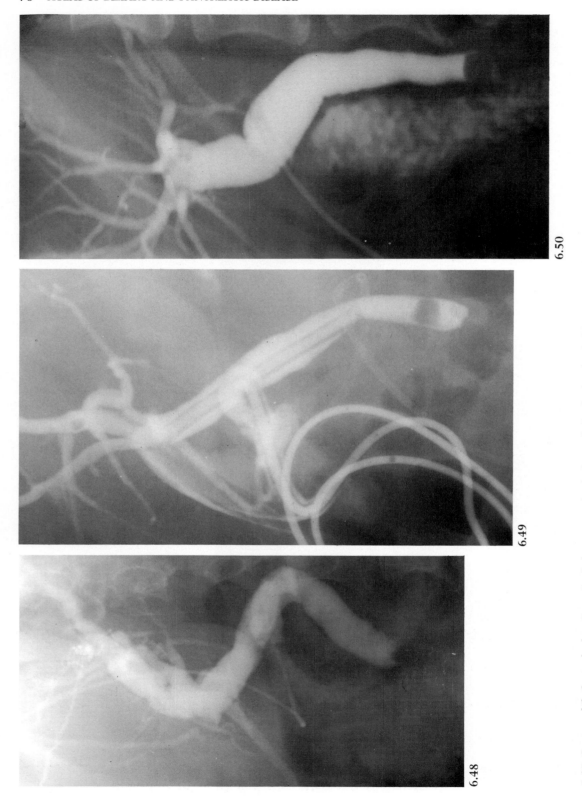

6.48 **Common bile duct calculus** *Operative cholangiogram* A calculus occludes the distal end of the common bile duct

6.49 **Choledocholithiasis** *T-tube cholangiogram* There are two calculi at the distal end of the common bile duct and a small one in the right posterior segment duct

6.50 **Choledocholithiasis** *T-tube cholangiogram* A single calculus is shown obstructing the distal end of the common bile duct. As a result, the bile ducts are distended and only a small amount of contrast medium is passing into the duodenum

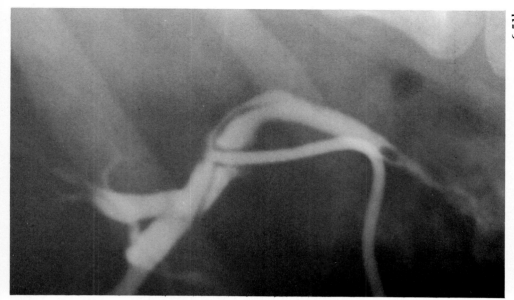

6.51b

6.51 **Bile duct calculus** *T-tube cholangiogram* a There is a sharply defined filling defect at the distal end of the common bile duct with some resulting delay in the passage of contrast medium into the duodenum. b A repeat examination carried out five days later shows it again, this time situated more proximally in the common bile duct. The size and shape remain unchanged, thus confirming that it is a calculus

6.51a

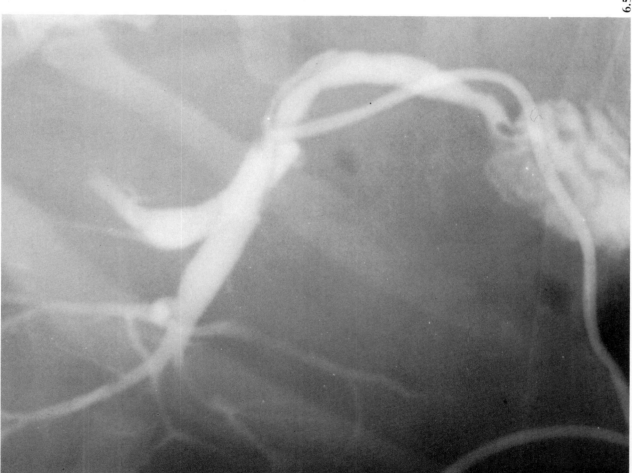

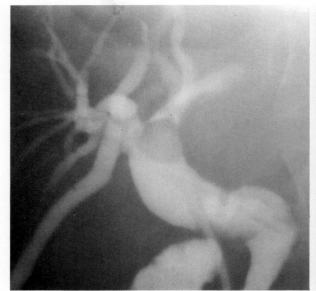

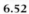
6.52

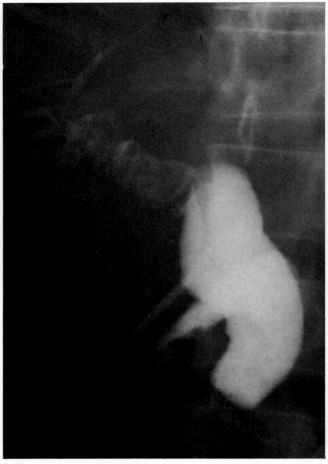
6.53

6.52 **Calculus in the common hepatic duct** *T-tube cholangiogram*
6.53 **Intrahepatic calculi in recurrent pyogenic cholangitis** (Wastie & Cunningham 1973) *T-tube cholangiogram* The common bile duct is dilated, and there is a stricture of the right hepatic duct with calculi above it. The left hepatic duct has not filled with contrast medium

Acute cholecystitis

In acute cholecystitis the gallbladder is usually enlarged and tense with areas of gangrenous necrosis, but free perforation is rare. The wall is characteristically thickened and oedematous and there is generally extensive inflammatory ulceration of the mucosa (Robbins & Angell 1976). More than 90 per cent. of cases result from impaction of a stone in Hartmann's pouch or in the cystic duct. Initially there is irritation of the gallbladder wall from the retained bile but bacterial inflammation is probably an integral part of the condition from the onset (Sherlock 1971).

The main presenting clinical feature is pain. This may begin as biliary colic but once inflammation becomes established the pain becomes well localized and sharp (Dawson 1973), and is made worse by movement of the abdominal wall and diaphragm. Nausea and vomiting are usual and some patients develop rigors; slight jaundice is sometimes present.

A diagnosis of acute cholecystitis is usually suspected on clinical grounds but infusion cholangiography is a useful investigation, particularly when early surgical intervention is being considered. A diagnosis of acute cholecystitis can be verified or regarded as highly probable in cases where the bile ducts are visualized but the gallbladder is not (Johnson *et al.* 1960; Becker *et al.* 1970). A film should be taken as late as four hours after the infusion of contrast medium before concluding that no gallbladder filling has occurred. Other conditions where the gallbladder fails to opacify include carcinoma of the gallbladder and strictures or oedema of the cystic duct, which are unlikely to present as acute abdominal emergencies. Narrowing and displacement of the bile ducts by the acutely inflamed gallbladder may be demonstrated at infusion cholangiography in patients with acute obstructive cholecystitis (Wise 1962; Nolan & Espiner 1972). These findings, when present, help to confirm the diagnosis.

References

Becker J., Borgström S., Fajers C.-M. & Saltzman G.-F. (1970) *Acta chir. scand.*, **136**, 197

Dawson J.L. (1973) *Clin. Gastroent.*, **2**, 85

Johnson H.C., McLaren J.R. & Weens H.S. (1960) *Radiology*, **74**, 790

Nolan D.J. & Espiner H.J. (1972) *Brit. J. Radiol.*, **45**, 821

Robbins S.L. & Angell M. (1976) *Basic Pathology*, Philadelpia: Saunders

Sherlock S. (1971) *Diseases of the Liver and Biliary System*. Oxford: Blackwell Scientific Publications

Wise R.E. (1962) *Intravenous Cholangiography*. Springfield, Illinois: Thomas

Acute emphysematous cholecystitis

Acute emphysematous cholecystitis is a rare form of acute cholecystitis in which gas is present in the lumen or the wall of the gallbladder, or in both, and also in the pericholecystic tissues. The first case was reported by Hegner in 1931 when a pre-operative diagnosis was made radiologically.

7 Cholecystitis

The aetiology of this condition is not fully understood. Gallbladder calculi and evidence of obstruction to the neck of the gallbladder were present in six of the seven patients operated on in one series (Rosoff & Meyers 1966) suggesting that the aetiology is similar to that of acute cholecystitis; the local tissue injury and ischaemia of the walls of the gallbladder which may accompany acute obstructive cholecystitis provides a favourable environment for the proliferation of dormant gas-producing bacteria in the gallbladder. As acute emphysematous cholecystitis is eight times more common in males, and 25 per cent. of patients are diabetic, May & Strong (1971) suggested that other aetiological factors must be involved. They found evidence to suggest that primary vascular occlusion of the cystic artery and its branches occurs and that the resulting ischaemia provides the conditions for the multiplication of micro-organisms present in the gallbladder. Vascular occlusion may account for the acute onset of the abdominal pain which is typical of this condition.

Fever and the sudden onset of intense right subcostal pain, similar to biliary colic, are the usual presenting clinical features.

The diagnosis is a radiological one and is made by observing the characteristic signs on a plain radiograph of the abdomen; these signs vary with the stage of the disease. The presence of gas in the gallbladder is shown as a mottled or homogeneous gas shadow in the right upper quadrant which conforms to the shape of the gallbladder (Blum & Stagg 1963). A fluid level is often present in the erect view and calculi are sometimes seen within the gallbladder shadow. The second stage of the disease is represented by a thin, concentric well-demarcated ring of gas in the wall of the gallbladder which later becomes streaked and bubble-like. A combination of gas in the lumen and wall of the gallbladder may be present and gas may also be present in the tissues around the gallbladder. Gas is not present in the bile ducts in acute emphysematous cholecystitis and this feature helps to differentiate it from biliary enteric fistulae and cholecyst-enterostomies.

The treatment is similar to that of acute cholecystitis beginning with intensive antibiotic therapy as soon as the diagnosis is made. Elective surgery can then be carried out at a later date when the condition of the patient permits (May & Strong 1971).

References

Blum L. & Stagg A. (1963) *Amer. J. Roentgenol.*, **89**, 840

Hegner C. F. (1931) *Arch. Surg.*, **22**, 993

McNulty J. G. (1977) *Radiology of the Liver*. London & Philadelphia: Saunders

May R. E. & Strong R. (1971) *Brit. J. Surg.*, **58**, 453

Rosoff L. & Meyers H. (1966) *Amer. J. Surg.*, **111**, 410

Chronic cholecystitis

Chronic cholecystitis is a common condition which may progress insidiously or develop following an attack of acute cholecystitis. The disease seems nearly always to be associated with cholelithiasis, unlike acute cholecystitis which may sometimes be acalculous (Lindberg *et al.* 1970).

The diagnosis is often difficult to make on clinical grounds alone as dyspepsia and poor tolerance of fatty foods are features of other digestive disorders as well as cholecystitis. Dull ache or localized tenderness may be present in the right hypochondrium and the temperature and white cell count are usually normal.

The principal pathological feature is thickening of the gallbladder wall which is due to hypertrophy of the muscle and mucosal layers initially, but which progresses to an atrophic stage with increasing inflammatory changes, mucosal destruction and sclerosis of the wall (Levine 1975). The result is a small, contracted viscus with an ulcerated mucosa and in advanced cases the gallbladder and cystic duct may shrink to form a fibrosed diverticulum of the common duct.

Chronic cholecystitis is usually associated with faint or absent opacification of the gallbladder during oral cholecystography, and re-examination with a doubled dose of contrast medium improves visualization in only a small proportion of patients. This may be because the lumen is filled with calculi, because the cystic duct is obstructed, because the gallbladder is poorly irrigated or because the diseased mucosa is unable to concentrate the contrast medium that does manage to enter the gallbladder. Failure of the gallbladder to contract after fat, during an otherwise normal cholecystogram, is a doubtful sign of gallbladder disease.

Intravenous cholangiography can show a shrunken gallbladder which has not been opacified by the oral technique, although filling may take longer than normal because of poor tidal flow of bile and contrast medium into the gallbladder. The major purpose of the examination is to demonstrate calculi. Suspected chronic cholecystitis is not an indication for retrograde cholangiography, but a contracted cavity may be shown incidentally, usually in patients with choledocholithiasis.

References

Levine T. (1975) *Chronic Cholecystitis*. New York: Halsted Press

Lindberg E. F., Grinnan G. L. B. & Smith L. (1970) *Ann. Surg.*, **171**, 152

Adenomyomatosis

This benign hyperplastic condition of the gallbladder wall is characterized by excessive proliferation of the surface epithelium and thickening of the muscle layer (Jutras &

Levesque 1966). The whole or part of the viscus may be involved and as a result three main varieties are recognized: the generalized type, the segmental type and the fundal type. In the normal gallbladder the Rokitansky–Aschoff sinuses do not penetrate as far as the muscularis and are regarded as normal structures, but in adenomyomatosis they are increased in number, depth and complexity with hyperplasia of the muscle layer (Colquhoun 1961). Dilated Rokitansky–Aschoff sinuses are often referred to as 'intramural diverticula'. Right upper quadrant pain, dyspepsia and fatty food intolerance are the usual presenting clinical features.

The diagnosis of adenomyomatosis is usually made at oral cholecystography. The generalized types show as a ring of dilated Rokitansky–Aschoff sinuses surrounding the gallbladder. These may only be evident on films taken half to three-quarters of an hour after a fatty meal. The segmental type usually produces strictures which are often single but may be multiple (Colquhoun 1961). Rokitansky–Aschoff sinuses may occur at the site of the stricture. A congenital fold extending across the lumen of the gallbladder, the 'Phrygian cap', may be confused with this variety of adenomyomatosis but the presence of Rokitansky–Aschoff sinuses on a film taken after gallbladder contraction differentiates adenomyomatosis from the Phrygian cap anomaly. In the fundal type there is a tumour-like thickening or a nodule at the fundus. Gallbladder calculi are often present in association with adenomyomatosis.

When gallbladders show evidence of strictures, septa, kinks, angular deformities or irregularities of outline, adenomyomatosis should be suspected and the films should be carefully examined for evidence of Rokitansky–Aschoff sinuses. Gallbladders which concentrate and contract well and contain calculi should also be suspect. Cholecystectomy has been said to give complete relief of symptoms (Ram & Midha 1975).

References

Colquhoun J. (1961) *Brit. J. Radiol.*, **34**, 101

Jutras J. A. & Levesque H.-P. (1966) *Radiol. Clin. N. Amer.*, **4**, 483

Ram M. D. & Midha D. (1975) *Surgery*, **78**, 224

Calcified gallbladder

Extensive calcification of the gallbladder wall, sometimes known as 'porcelain gallbladder' is associated with few symptoms and is often discovered as an incidental finding on abdominal radiographs. It is an uncommon condition, the cause of which is unknown, but it is believed that chronic cystic duct obstruction causes large quantities of calcium carbonate to pass from the wall of the gallbladder into its lumen. In this way calcification of the gallbladder wall occurs as well as an increase of calcium salts in the lumenal contents (Phemister *et al.* 1931; Cornell & Clarke 1959). Gallstones are present in nearly all cases of gallbladder calcification and usually a stone obstructs the cystic duct. The gallbladder wall is usually thickened and low grade chronic inflammation is also considered to play a part in the aetiology. It has been postulated that localized calcification of the gallbladder can result from calcification of cholesterol plaques.

The appearance of calcification in the wall of the gallbladder is seen on the radiograph as linear, flaky or plaque-like calcification in the expected position of the gallbladder (Ochsner & Carrera 1963). The calcification also takes the shape of the gallbladder and this should suggest the correct diagnosis. Oblique and lateral views are usually decisive.

Carcinoma occurs in the porcelain gallbladder with sufficient frequency to warrant prophylactic cholecystectomy even when the disease is asymptomatic (Berk *et al.* 1973).

References

Berk R. N., Armbuster T. G. & Saltzstein S. L. (1973) *Radiology*, **106**, 29

Cornell C. M. & Clarke R. (1959) *Ann. Surg.*, **149**, 267

Ochsner S. F. & Carrera G. M. (1963) *Amer. J. Roentgenol.*, **89**, 847

Phemister D. B., Rewbridge A. G. & Rudishill H. Jnr. (1931) *J. Amer. med. Ass.*, **97**, 1843

Limy bile

Chronic partial obstruction of the cystic duct, usually by a calculus, may cause large quantities of calcium carbonate to pass into the lumen of the gallbladder and as a result the gallbladder contents may show as radiopaque fluid on radiographs of the abdomen. The condition is known as 'limy bile' or 'milk of calcium bile'. Gallstones are almost always present in the gallbladder in this condition. Spontaneous passage of limy bile and associated gallstones is not uncommon and the limy bile may completely disappear (Holden & Turner 1972)

Reference

Holden W. S. & Turner M. J. (1972) *Clin. Radiol.*, **23**, 500

Cholesterosis of the gallbladder

Cholesterosis of the gallbladder occurs in two forms, diffuse or localized (Feldman & Feldman 1954). In the diffuse form the mucous membrane is congested, reddened and covered with small lipid deposits; it is also known as 'strawberry gallbladder'. Radiographs of the gallbladder appear normal and cholecystography is usually unhelpful in making the diagnosis.

In the localized form of cholesterosis, the lipid deposits are heaped up to form papillomatous outgrowths that are usually present around the neck of the gallbladder. In this form the concentration of the contrast medium in the gallbladder is usually normal and the characteristic appearance is the presence of single or multiple small filling defects fixed to the gallbladder wall. Tangental views may show the filling defect arising from the wall (Samuel & Komins 1957).

References

Feldman M. & Feldman M. Jnr. (1954) *Gastroenterology*, **27**, 641

Samuel E. & Komins C. (1957) *Brit. J. Radiol.*, **30**, 356

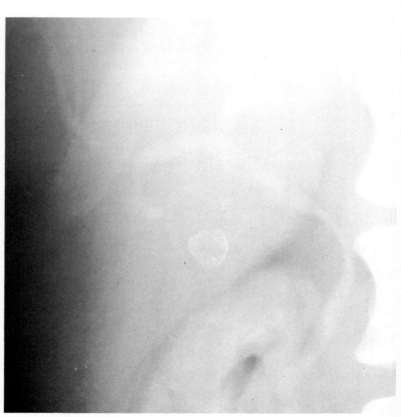

7.1

7.1 **Acute cholecystitis** *Infusion cholangiogram* The gallbladder did not fill with contrast medium. The bile ducts are visualized and a segment of the common bile duct is narrowed with medial convexity and displacement due to compression from the acutely inflamed and distended gallbladder. A radiopaque calculus is present in the non-visualized gallbladder

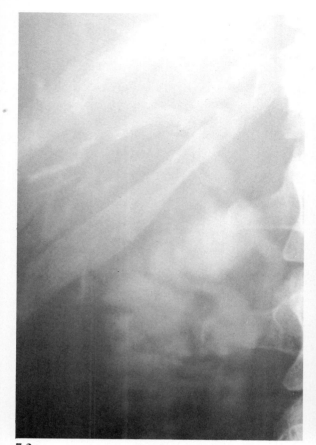

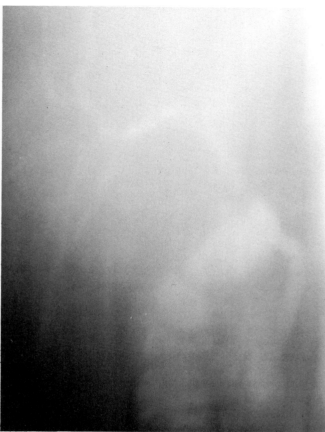

7.2a

7.2b

7.2 **Acute cholecystitis** *Infusion cholangiography with tomography* a, b There is marked upward displacement and convexity with narrowing of the hepatic duct due to compression from an acutely inflamed and distended gallbladder which has not opacified

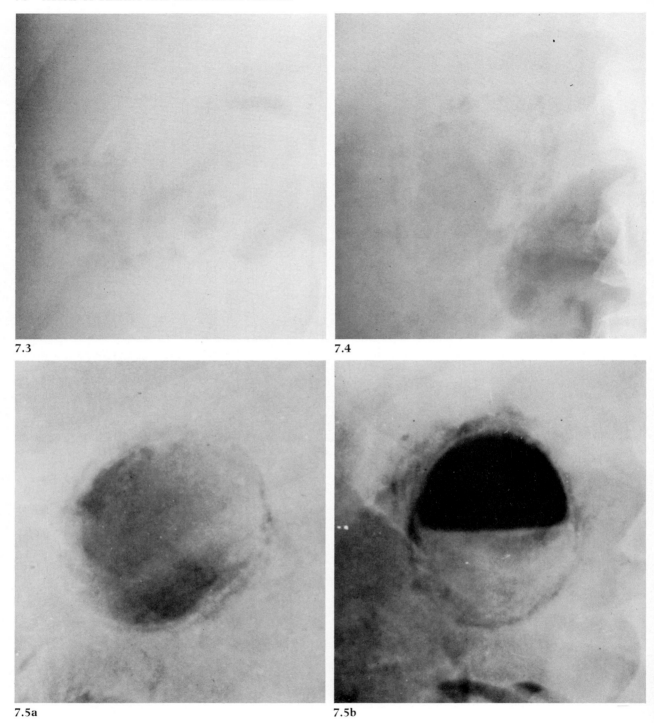

7.3

7.4

7.5a

7.5b

7.3 **Acute emphysematous cholecystitis** *Plain film* An irregular mottled gas shadow is shown in the right upper quadrant
7.4 **Acute emphysematous cholecystitis** *Plain film* Gas is present in the lumen and wall of the gallbladder
7.5 **Acute emphysematous cholecystitis** (May & Strong 1971) *Plain film of abdomen* a The gallbladder is outlined by a thin halo of radiolucency surrounding the main gas shadow. b In the erect view a fluid level is present in the gas-filled gallbladder

7.6 Acute emphysematous cholecystitis *Plain film* Gas is present in the wall of the gallbladder (McNulty 1977)
7.7 Chronic cholecystitis *Retrograde cholangiogram* The gallbladder is small and irregular in outline
7.8 Adenomyomatosis *Oral cholecystogram* A ring of Rokitansky–Aschoff sinuses containing contrast medium surrounds the gallbladder on the film taken after a fatty meal (Courtesy of Prof. J.H. Middlemiss)

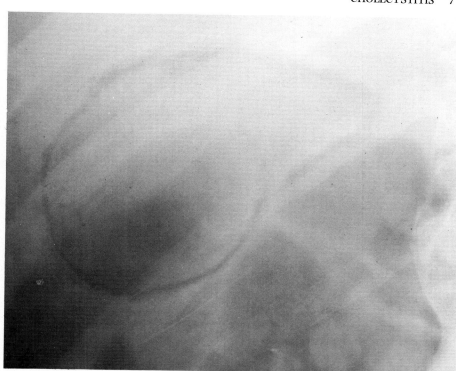

7.6

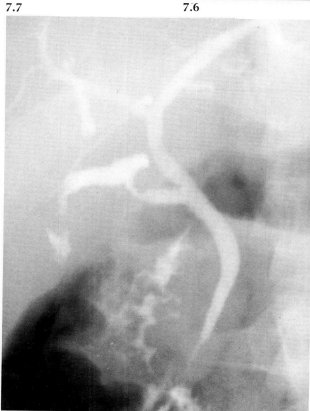

7.7

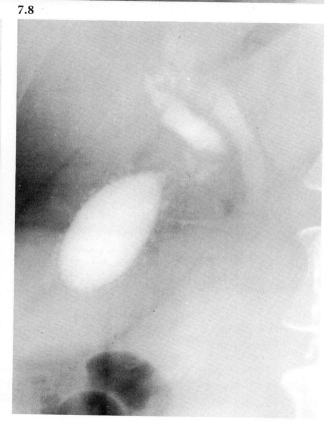

7.8

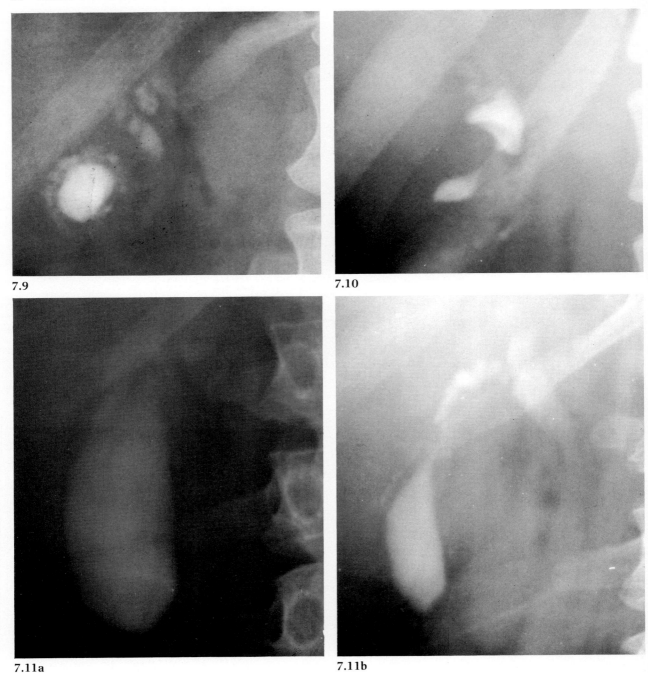

7.9

7.10

7.11a   7.11b

7.9 Adenomyomatosis *Oral cholecystogram* Marked gallbladder contraction has occurred after a fatty meal. A ring of large Rokitansky–Aschoff sinuses surrounds the gallbladder (Courtesy of Prof. J.H. Middlemiss)

7.10 Adenomyomatosis *Oral cholecystogram* There is a stricture and marked thickening of the gallbladder wall. A small number of Rokitansky–Aschoff sinuses are outlined with contrast medium

7.11 Adenomyomatosis *Oral cholecystogram* a The gallbladder appears normal apart from slight irregularity of the fundus.
b *Film taken after fat.* The gallbladder has contracted well and there are Rokitansky–Aschoff sinuses throughout the gallbladder. This examination emphasizes the importance of the fatty meal in making the diagnosis of adenomyomatosis

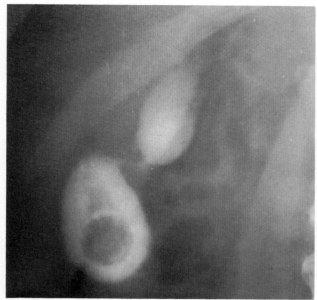

7.13

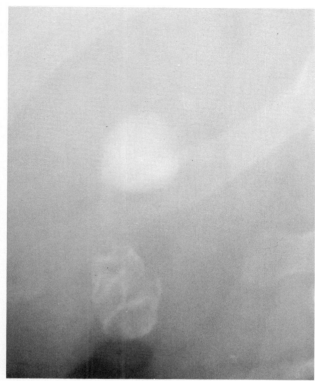

7.12

7.14

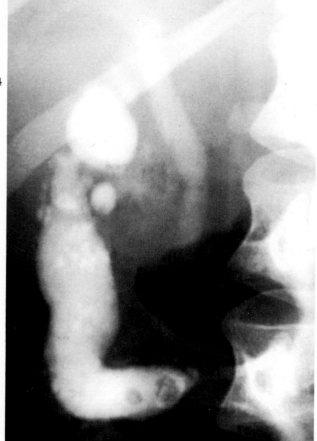

7.12 Adenomyomatosis *Oral cholecystogram* There is a
stricture of the body of the gallbladder and several calculi are
imprisoned within the fundus
7.13 Adenomyomatosis *Oral cholecystogram* There is a
stricture of the body of the gallbladder and calculi are present
in the fundus which is irregular in outline
7.14 Adenomyomatosis *Infusion cholangiogram* There is a
stricture of the neck of the gallbladder and two radiolucent
calculi are present in the fundus. Rokitansky–Aschoff sinuses
filled with contrast medium are shown extending beyond the
lumen and as denser opacities overlying the body of the
gallbladder

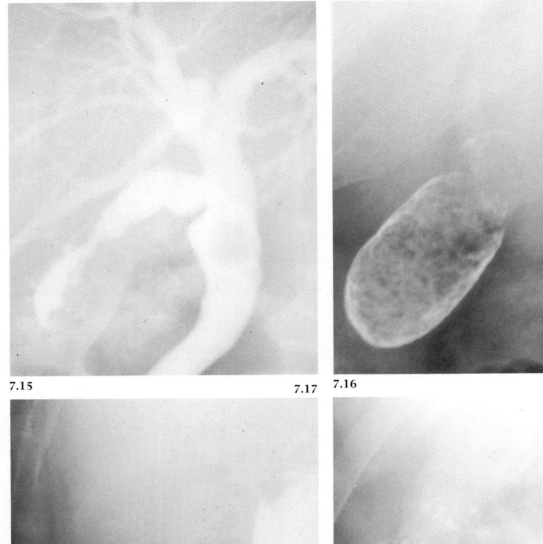

7.15

7.16

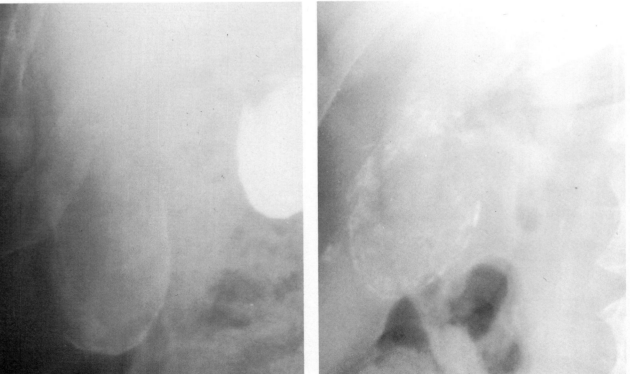

7.17

7.18

Opposite page
7.15 **Adenomyomatosis** *Retrograde cholangiogram* The gallbladder is contracted, with filling of Rokitansky–Aschoff sinuses within its thickened wall. There is also a calculus in the common bile duct
7.16 **Porcelain gallbladder** *Plain film* Extensive calcification is present in the wall of the gallbladder
7.17 **Porcelain gallbladder** *Barium meal* Calcification in the wall of the gallbladder was noted during a barium examination
7.18 **Calcified gallbladder** *Plain film* There is patchy calcification in the wall of the gallbladder

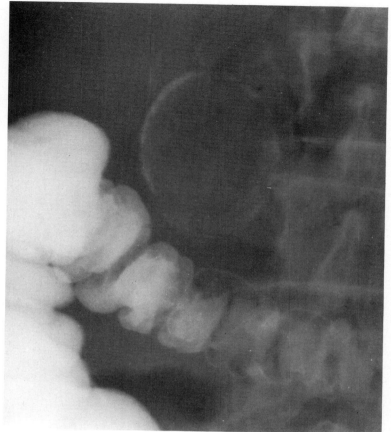

7.19a

7.19b

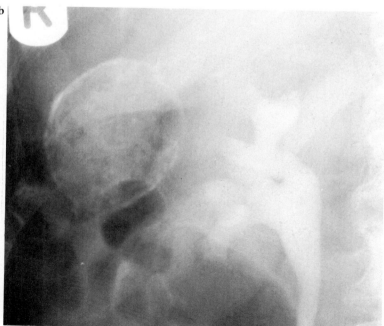

7.19 **Porcelain gallbladder** *Barium enema* a An oval calcified opacity was noted at barium enema examination. The possibility of this being a renal mass was considered but b an urographic examination showed that it was not related to the right kidney and the correct diagnosis of a calcified gallbladder was made

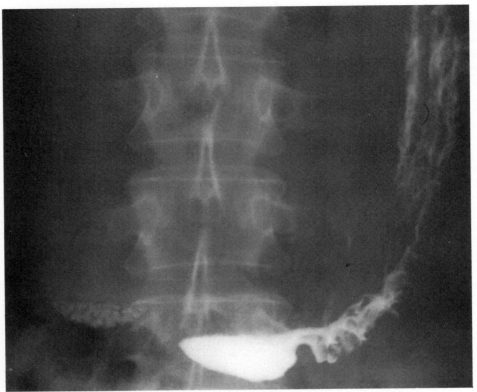

7.20 **Limy bile and cholelithiasis** *Barium meal* There is faint opacification of the gallbladder by limy bile. Multiple small radiopaque calculi are also present

7.21 **Limy bile and cholelithiasis** *Plain abdomen* Multiple large radiolucent gallbladder calculi are outlined by limy bile

7.22 **Limy bile and cholelithiasis** *Plain film* A preliminary film taken prior to excretion urography shows multiple calculi in the gallbladder which is well opacified by limy bile. There is also a calculus present in the cystic duct

7.20

7.21

7.22

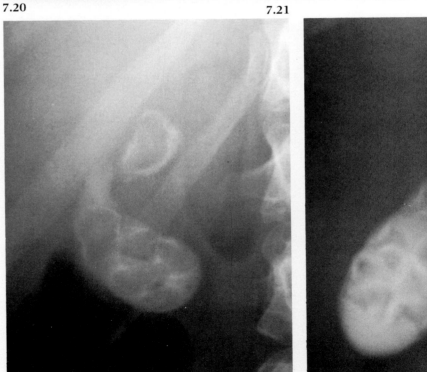

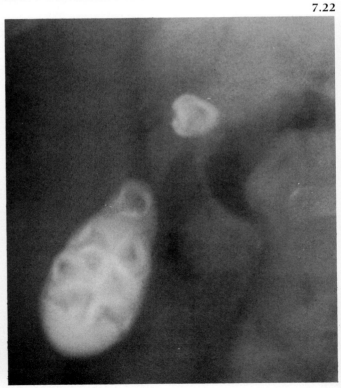

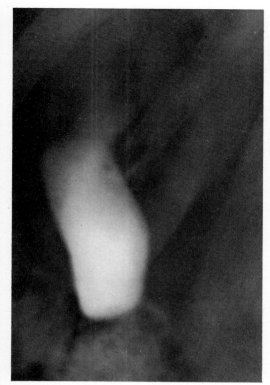

7.23a

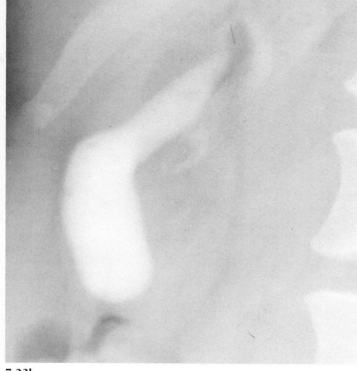

7.23b

7.24

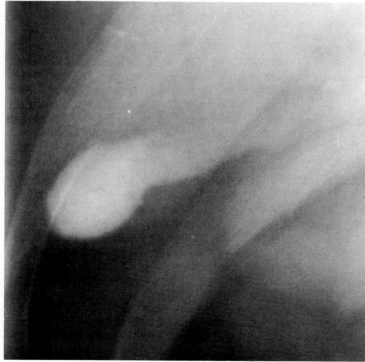

7.23 Papillomatous cholesterosis of the gallbladder *Oral cholecystogram* a There is good opacification of the gallbladder and some filling defects are present in the neck of the gallbladder. b The filling defects are better seen on the film taken after a fatty meal and show no change in position in different views

7.24 Papillomatous cholesterosis *Oral cholecystogram (film taken after fat)* The outline of the gallbladder is slightly irregular and filling defects are present in the body and neck of the gallbladder

8 Benign Biliary Stricture

Papillary stenosis

The commonest cause of stenosis at the lower end of the common bile duct is duct calculus, when infection and damage from stones cause fibrosis and scarring in the sphincteric region. The resulting strictures may be localized adjacent to the papilla and produce dilatation of the common bile duct or they may be more extensive and also involve the intrapancreatic bile duct. Stricturing in the sphincteric region may result from the use of metal dilators during surgical exploration of the common bile duct (Thorbjarnarson 1975). Whether papillary or sphincteric fibrosis and stenosis may occur as a primary condition in the absence of bile duct calculi is a subject of controversy, since it is possible that an offending calculus may lacerate the sphincter during its passage (Nardi & Acosta 1966). Certainly, papillary stenosis may be present when no calculus can be found in the common duct and when no previous duct exploration has been performed.

The symptomatology in patients with papillary stenosis may be vague. Most often there is persistence of pain following cholecystectomy; there may be mild jaundice with elevation of the alkaline phosphatase level and intravenous cholangiography may provide evidence of dilatation of the common bile duct. A common bile duct width of 12 mm may be regarded as the normal upper limit in a young subject although 14 mm would be more appropriate in a large or elderly patient. Such dilatation need not imply papillary stenosis since there may be residual dilatation following surgical removal of common duct calculi. Small impacted sphincteric calculi may not be evident on the intravenous cholangiogram but may produce delayed emptying into the duodenum; endoscopic cholangiography can give better delineation of the sphincteric region and can better exclude the possibility of small calculi. Operative radiomanometry prior to surgical exploration of the duct has been recommended in the diagnosis of papillary stenosis (White *et al.* 1972).

Endoscopic biliary manometry is unsatisfactory because the presence of a catheter in the sphincter may induce sphincteric contraction and delay emptying.

Biliary dyskinesia is a title which implies an abnormality of sphincteric function which is associated with painful symptoms, but as normal sphincteric function is so hard to assess, this is a difficult entity to evaluate. Contraction of an otherwise normal biliary sphincter with delayed but dramatic emptying after 10 minutes may be observed during endoscopic cholangiography. The situation is hardly physiological since there has been sphincteric cannulation and the common bile duct is filled with hypertonic contrast medium.

References

Nardi G.L. & Acosta J.M. (1966) *Ann. Surg.*, **164**, 611

Thorbjarnarson B. (1975) *Surgery of the Biliary Tract*. Philadelphia: Saunders

White T.T., Waisman H., Hopton D. & Kavlie H. (1972) *Amer. J. Surg.*, **123**, 73

Benign stricture of the common bile duct

The majority of fibrous strictures of the common duct develop following cholecystectomy, although blunt abdominal trauma and gastric surgery may also be responsible. Deepening jaundice in the post-cholecystectomy period will arouse suspicion that the extrahepatic bile duct has been ligated and a profuse discharge of bile might indicate an incision or tear. In a small proportion of patients obstruction may not be evident until months or years after cholecystectomy (Smith 1975). Bouts of intermittent fever due to associated cholangitis may occur. The extrahepatic bile duct may become involved by the clamps and ligatures used to achieve haemostasis, or the use of excessive traction may bring a portion of the common duct into the cystic duct ligature. Subhepatic pooling of bile is a sequel to tearing or crushing of the bile duct and although it has been implicated as a cause of periductal fibrosis and stricture it is more likely that preceding trauma to the duct is responsible.

Although commonly sited at the level of the cystic duct entrance into the common duct, many fibrous strictures occur at a higher level, leaving less than a centimetre of patent common hepatic duct below the liver. Direct cholangiography by either the endoscopic or percutaneous approaches is of most value in defining the level and character of a stricture. If bile ducts above the stricture are not clearly outlined at endoscopic retrograde cholangiography the percutaneous method must then be used, as knowledge of the anatomy of the proximal ducts is so important in planning surgical repair (George et al. 1965). Where it is available the endoscopic method should be used first, because the risk of bile leakage and the need for prompt surgical exploration are minimized, and in the majority of subjects will provide all the necessary information. Since these patients are often markedly jaundiced, intravenous cholangiography is usually unhelpful. Antibiotic cover is recommended for both methods of direct cholangiography.

In patients who become jaundiced several years after cholecystectomy it may be hard to decide between post-operative stricture and bile duct carcinoma. Traumatic strictures tend to be smooth and may be only a few millimetres in length whereas malignant strictures are characteristically elongated, irregular and associated with shouldered or polypoid filling defects on the cholangiogram; however, extensive fibrosis may produce elongation of a stricture which may be hard to distinguish from sclerosing bile duct carcinoma. Histological examination of surgical biopsies may also be indecisive in these circumstances.

Though designated benign, traumatic bile duct strictures are associated with a high mortality rate in excess of 10 per cent. (Warren & Jefferson 1973); the prognosis is determined by the adequacy of surgical repair, the length of the period of obstruction and the presence of secondary biliary cirrhosis.

References

George P., Young W.B., Walker J.G. & Sherlock S. (1965) *Brit. J. Surg.*, **52**, 779

Smith R. (1975) *Surgery of the Liver, Pancreas and Biliary Tract*, p. 165 (Ed. Najarian J.S. & Delaney J.P.). New York: Stratton Intercontinental Medical Book Corporation

Warren K.W. & Jefferson M.F. (1973) *Surg. Clin. N. Amer.*, **53**, 1169

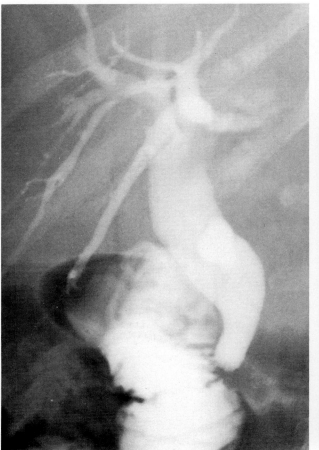

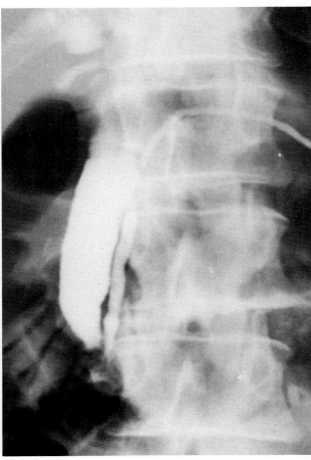

8.1

8.2

8.1 **Papillary stenosis** A 42-year-old woman with persistent pain and bouts of jaundice following cholecystectomy one year previously *Endoscopic cholangiogram* The extrahepatic ducts and cystic duct remnant are dilated above a constantly narrowed sphincter. The common hepatic duct measures 2·5 cm in diameter. Emptying of contrast medium into the duodenum was delayed. No calculi are present

8.2 **Papillary stenosis** A middle-aged woman with vague upper abdominal pain for two years following cholecystectomy *Endoscopic cholangiogram and pancreatogram* The common bile duct is dilated above the papilla and measures 1·9 cm in diameter. Drainage of contrast medium into the duodenum was delayed. No calculi are present

Opposite page

8.3 **Biliary dyskinesia** A sensible 65-year-old man experienced persistent upper abdominal pain following cholecystectomy for gallbladder stones nine months previously; the pain was identical to that experienced prior to operation. Operative cholangiography had shown no bile duct stones *Endoscopic cholangiogram* a Following withdrawal of the endoscope, the common bile duct has lost its normal tapered configuration and is 1·5 cm in diameter. The cystic duct remnant is distended. No contrast medium entered the duodenum for about 5 minutes until b the sphincter relaxed and allowed it to enter the duodenum and reflux into the pancreatic duct. The cannulation of the bile duct was relatively easy and there had been no trauma to the papilla. The later films show that there was no fibrotic stenosis of the sphincter

8.4 **Papillary stenosis** A middle-aged woman with upper abdominal pain and jaundice *Endoscopic cholangiogram* There are small lucent stones in the gallbladder and upper common bile duct. The intrahepatic bile ducts are dilated. The common bile duct is dilated above the sphincter, is irregular in outline and has lost the normal tapered configuration. There was delayed emptying of contrast medium into the duodenum

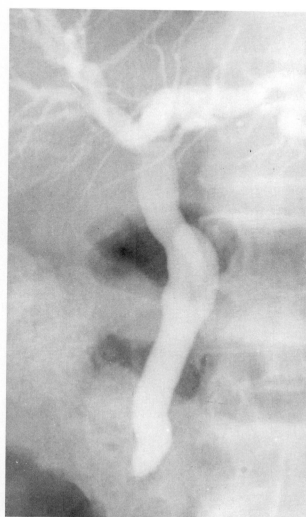

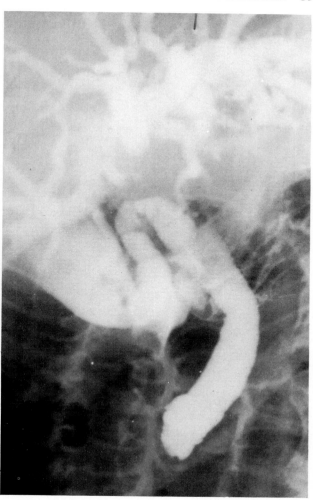

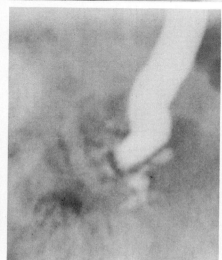

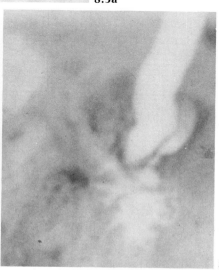

8.3a

8.4

8.3b

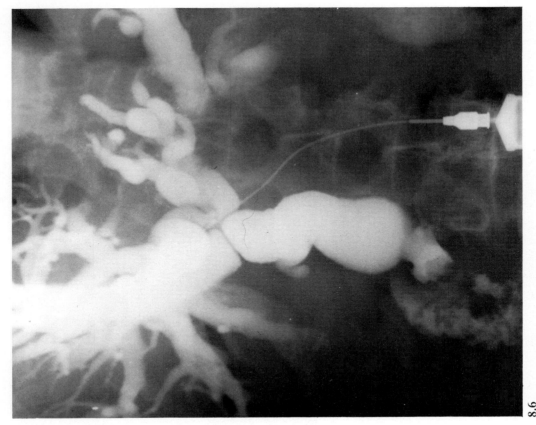

8.6

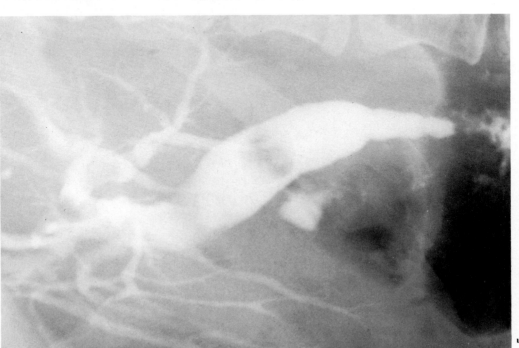

8.5

8.5 **Benign strictures of the lower common bile duct associated with bile duct calculus** *Endoscopic cholangiogram* The common duct is dilated above two short strictures in the lower common bile duct within which lies a large radiolucent calculus. A further radiolucent calculus is present in the left lateral segment duct. Cholecystectomy had been performed

8.6 **Benign stricture associated with bile duct calculus** A 52-year-old woman with a two-week history of jaundice and a previous cholecystectomy *Percutaneous cholangiogram* A large radiolucent stone lies at the lower end of the common bile duct with a stricture above it. At operation the lower common bile duct was grossly thickened (Courtesy of Dr. G. Evison)

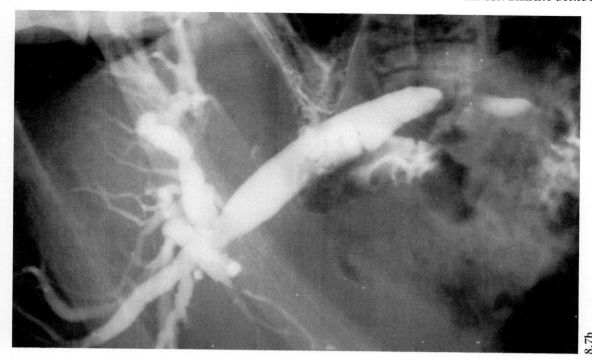

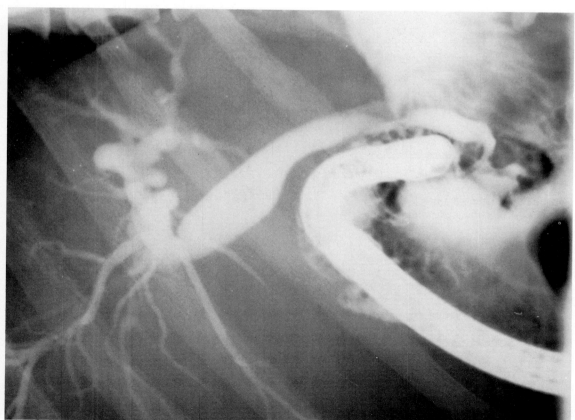

8.7a

8.7b

8.7 Stricture of the common bile duct following cholecystectomy *Endoscopic cholangiogram* a There is a short strictured region of the common bile duct 4 cm above the papilla. The common hepatic duct is dilated. b Following withdrawal of the endoscope contrast medium was held up in the common duct above the stricture

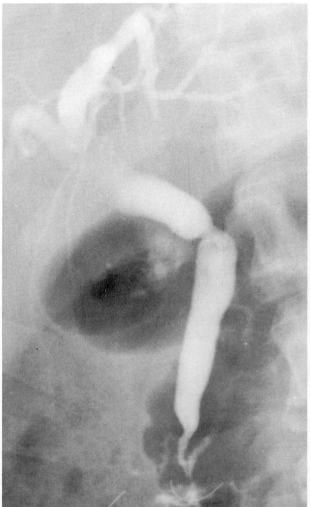

8.8

8.9

8.10

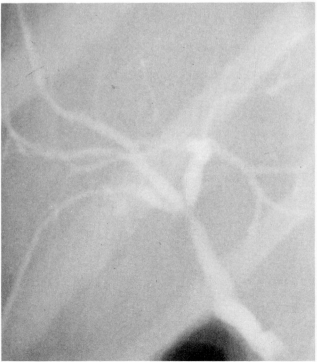

8.8 **Post-operative stricture of the common hepatic duct** Young woman with persistent mild jaundice which developed following an apparently uneventful cholecystectomy six months previously *Endoscopic cholangiogram* There is a short cystic duct remnant and a stricture of the common hepatic duct 1 cm above its insertion into the main duct. The position of the stricture suggests that the duct may have been damaged during vascular ligation

8.9 **Post-operative stricture of the common hepatic duct** A 29-year-old woman experienced bouts of mild jaundice in the year following cholecystectomy for gallbladder stones. Operative cholangiography or exploration of the bile ducts were not performed *Endoscopic cholangiogram* A stricture of the common hepatic duct is seen at the confluence of the intrahepatic ducts, well above the cystic duct. Pooling of irritant bile adjacent to the confluence following operation has been advanced as the cause for such high post-operative strictures

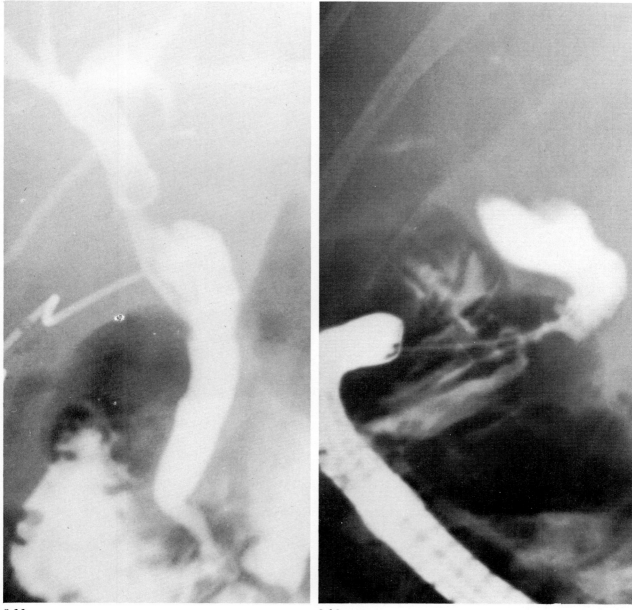

8.11   **8.12**

8.11 **Post-operative stricture of the common duct** *T-tube cholangiogram* Immediate post-operative demonstration of a stricture of the common hepatic duct adjacent to the cystic duct insertion, with a calculus above it. Such a stricture may be due to excessive traction on the cystic duct whereby a portion of the main duct wall becomes involved in the cystic duct ligature

8.12 **Post-operative stricture of the common bile duct** *Endoscopic cholangiogram* The common bile duct is obstructed 4 cm above the papilla

(Opposite page)

8.10   **Post-operative stricture of the common hepatic duct** A 52-year-old woman with jaundice and febrile episodes for four months who had had a cholecystectomy 10 years previously. A fibrotic stricture was confirmed at laparotomy *Endoscopic cholangiogram* A stricture of the common hepatic duct is seen at the level of the confluence of the intrahepatic ducts, which are slightly dilated

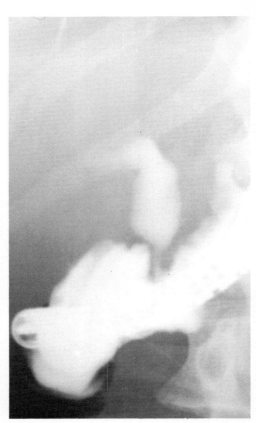

8.14

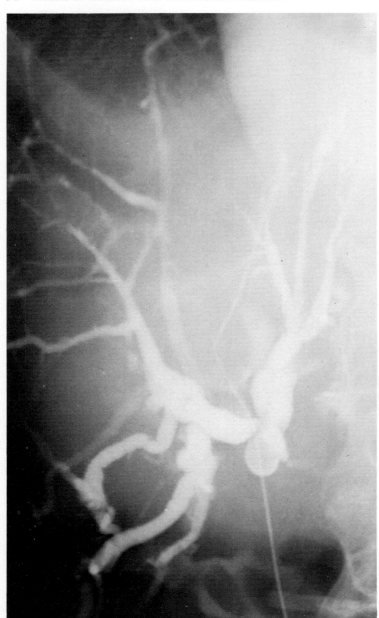

8.13

8.13 **Post-operative stricture of the common bile duct** A 72-year-old woman whose common hepatic duct was damaged at cholecystectomy three years previously. An inflammatory stricture was demonstrated at laparotomy *Percutaneous cholangiogram* The intrahepatic ducts are dilated above a stricture of the common hepatic duct, and a calculus is to be seen proximal to the stricture (Courtesy of Dr. G. Evison)

8.14 **Stricture at choledochoduodenostomy** A choledochoduodenostomy had been performed several years previously *Endoscopic cholangiogram* The stoma was cannulated. There is a 1 cm stricture of the common bile duct which is dilated proximally

Primary sclerosing cholangitis

9 Cholangitis

Primary sclerosing cholangitis is characterized by non-specific inflammatory fibrosis in the submucosa of the biliary tree, with constriction of the extrahepatic and intrahepatic ducts giving a thickened cord-like appearance (Thompson & Read 1974). The condition may occur in association with a number of disorders of which ulcerative colitis is the most common (Smith & Loe 1965). Other associations which have been described include Crohn's disease, retroperitoneal fibrosis, Riedel's thyroiditis (Bartholomew *et al.* 1963), and chronic pancreatitis (Waldram *et al.* 1975).

The disorder, which occurs most commonly in men, usually presents with progressive obstructive jaundice; loss of weight and vague upper abdominal pain are common. Mitochondrial antibodies are generally absent from the serum, so excluding primary biliary cirrhosis, and liver biopsy may show a characteristic onion skin pattern of fibrous tissue around the bile ducts. The diagnosis of primary sclerosing cholangitis can be suggested if a patient develops progressive obstructive jaundice without a history of previous biliary surgery or bile duct calculi and if there is generalized thickening and stenosis of the biliary system. Sclerosing bile duct carcinoma should have been excluded by laparotomy and biopsy or prolonged follow-up.

Intravenous cholangiography is usually ineffective in demonstrating the biliary tree and endoscopic cholangiography is the investigation of choice. Percutaneous cholangiography is relatively unsuccessful because puncture of the narrowed intrahepatic ducts is difficult. Retrograde cholangiography may demonstrate beaded narrowing of the intrahepatic and extrahepatic ducts, including the cystic duct, although contrast medium may not pass retrogradely into the intrahepatic ducts because of obstruction. Multiple biliary strictures and beading are often patchily distributed and there may be pruning of intrahepatic duct radicles. If a long stricture is shown, sclerosing cholangiocarcinoma must be considered (Thorpe *et al.* 1967).

Endoscopic cholangiography can be used to monitor the progress of the disease during conservative management as there is some evidence that steroid therapy may have a favourable effect.

References

Bartholomew L.G., Cain J.C., Woolner L.B., Utz D.C. & Ferris D.O. (1963) *New Engl. J. Med.*, **269**, 8

Burwood R.J., Davies G.T., Lawrie B.W., Blumgart L.H. & Salmon P.R. (1973) *Clin. Radiol.*, **24**, 397

Smith M.P. & Loe R.H. (1965) *Amer. J. Surg.*, **110**, 239

Thompson B.W. & Read R.C. (1974) *Amer. J. Surg.*, **128**, 777

Thorpe M.E.C., Scheuer P.J. & Sherlock S. (1967) *Gut*, **8**, 435

Waldram R., Kopelman H., Tsantoulas D. & Williams R. (1975) *Lancet*, **i**, 550

Infective cholangitis

Bacterial infection of the bile is found in most cases of calculous disease of the bile ducts and biliary stricture (Scott & Khan 1967). Infective cholangitis may have either an acute or chronic clinical course and is usually associated with partial biliary obstruction due to choledocholithiasis or stricture. Rarely, neoplastic obstruction may be the primary lesion. Infective cholangitis may supervene in patients with cystic dilatation of the intrahepatic bile ducts.

Acute infective cholangitis Shivering, increasing pain and jaundice may develop in acute cholangitis as mucosal oedema completes bile duct obstruction. Acute obstructive cholangitis may be associated with liver abscesses, and unless cholangitis is adequately treated it may be complicated by Gram-negative septicaemia, shock and renal failure. The introduction of contrast medium into the biliary tree by either percutaneous or retrograde cholangiography may provoke complications so that these investigations are contraindicated in patients with acute cholangitis.

Chronic infective cholangitis If infective cholangitis is prolonged, widespread fibrosis of the extrahepatic bile ducts and stricturing of the intrahepatic ducts may occur, owing to bile leakage and the formation of periductal abscesses. Biliary cirrhosis and portal hypertension will develop if obstruction persists.

Endoscopic cholangiography is the method of choice for demonstrating the obstructing lesion because excretion of intravenous contrast medium is impaired. Adequate antibiotic cover is most important. Excessive amounts of hypertonic contrast medium injected above the obstructing stone or stricture may produce chemical cholangitis and provoke acute infective cholangitis so that the minimum amount of medium necessary to demonstrate the cause of obstruction should be used. The risk of provoking acute exacerbation in patients with chronic cholangitis is greater with percutaneous cholangiography, especially with the fine needle technique since in this method the obstructed ducts cannot be decompressed, and the pressure within them is raised when contrast medium is injected.

Stricturing of the extrahepatic ducts may extend to involve the intrahepatic ducts and give them a beaded appearance which is due to dilatation of the ducts between multiple short strictures. The ducts may also present a finely irregular outline on the cholangiogram.

Recurrent pyogenic cholangitis (Oriental cholangitis) Pyogenic cholangitis associated with gross dilatation of intrahepatic and extrahepatic bile ducts which contain biliary mud, soft pigment stones and pus occurs quite commonly in Japan, Malaya, Singapore and Hong Kong (Wastie & Cunningham 1973). The condition is characterized by intermittent biliary fever, sometimes with repeated attacks over several years which may terminate in acute liver failure or culminate in biliary cirrhosis (Ong & Kong 1962). Infestation of the bile ducts with the liver fluke *Clonorchis sinesis* complicated with an *Escherichia coli*

infection has been suggested as the cause of this condition, but Clonorchis does not occur in Malaya where pyogenic cholangitis is prevalent.

Intravenous cholangiography gives limited diagnostic information and the best delineation of the biliary tree has been achieved by operative and T-tube cholangiography. Strictures, stones and dilatation of the intrahepatic and extrahepatic bile ducts are the most striking radiological features. It is interesting that although all the hepatic ducts may be involved in some patients, the ducts in the right lobe are those most likely to be spared (Wastie & Cunningham 1973).

References
Ong G. B. & Kong, H. (1962) *Arch. Surg.*, **84**, 199

Scott A. J. & Khan G. A. (1967) *Lancet*, **ii**, 790

Wastie M. L. & Cunningham I. G. E. (1973) *Amer. J. Roentgenol.*, **119**, 71

Hydatid disease

Man may act as the intermediate host in the cycle of the tapeworm *Echinococcus granulosa*, which lives in dogs, but hydatid disease occurs commonly in association with sheep rearing, as sheep also act as intermediate hosts. The liver is the common site for the development of hydatid cysts, although the lungs, spleen, brain and bones may be affected. Mediterranean and Middle Eastern countries have the highest incidence.

Rupture of hydatid cysts into the bile ducts may lead to spontaneous cure or to obstructive jaundice with cholangitis or liver abscess (Zielinski & Elmslie 1969). Although eosinophilia may be a feature, the Casoni or hydatid complement fixation tests are usually positive.

Hepatic hydatid cysts may produce enlargement of the liver with elevation of the right hemidiaphragm. Calcification may occur in the ectocyst and be evident as mural calcification on the plain abdominal radiograph. Hepatic scintigraphy is of great value in demonstrating defects within the liver which may be shown by ultrasonic examination to contain fluid. Ruptured cysts within the extrahepatic bile ducts may be demonstrated at endoscopic retrograde or operative cholangiography, but if hydatid disease is suspected, percutaneous cholangiography is contraindicated, because of the risks of anaphylactic reaction and implantation of daughter cysts.

Reference
Zielinski V. E. & Elmslie R. G. (1969) *Med. J. Aust.*, **1**, 839

Ascariasis

Roundworm infestation is extremely common in many

tropical countries and involvement of the biliary tract may occur (Pfeffermann *et al.* 1972). Though the worms are large they may find their way through the duodenal papilla into the common bile duct and dead worms may become calcified to form bile duct calculi. Patients present with jaundice, evidence of cholangitis or liver abscess. Intravenous cholangiography shows evidence of bile duct obstruction in 75 per cent. of patients, and linear filling defects due to the worms may be evident (Cremin 1969). Cholangiography may be repeated following the use of a vermifuge, though surgical treatment is usually necessary.

References

Cremin B. J. (1969) *Brit. J. Radiol.*, **42**, 506

Pfeffermann R., Floman Y. & Rozin R. R. (1972) *Arch. Surg.*, **105**, 118

Clonorchiasis

The Chinese liver fluke *Clonorchis sinensis* is found mainly in eastern Asia, but is also seen in emigrants from China in other parts of the world. The flukes reside in the bile ducts where they provoke intermittent biliary obstruction and recurrent pyogenic cholangitis following which they may perish (Cremin 1969). There is some doubt as to whether Clonorchis infestation is the invariable cause of oriental pyogenic cholangitis (Wastie & Cunningham 1973).

The parasites are seen as linear arch-shaped lucencies at percutaneous and operative cholangiography, but are rarely shown by intravenous cholangiography (Okuda *et al.* 1973).

References

Cremin B. J. (1969) *Brit. J. Radiol.*, **42**, 506

Okuda K., Emura T., Morokuma K., Kojima S. & Yokagawa M. (1973) *Gastroenterology*, **65**, 457

Wastie M. L. & Cunningham I. G. E. (1973) *Amer. J. Roentgenol.*, **119**, 71

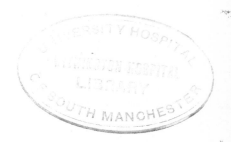

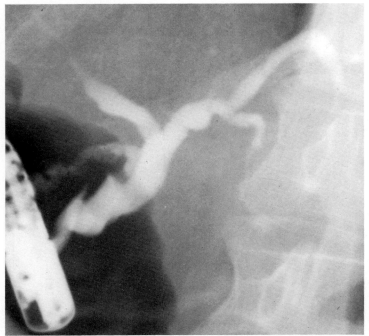

9.1

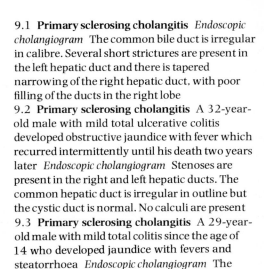

9.1 **Primary sclerosing cholangitis** *Endoscopic cholangiogram* The common bile duct is irregular in calibre. Several short strictures are present in the left hepatic duct and there is tapered narrowing of the right hepatic duct, with poor filling of the ducts in the right lobe

9.2 **Primary sclerosing cholangitis** A 32-year-old male with mild total ulcerative colitis developed obstructive jaundice with fever which recurred intermittently until his death two years later *Endoscopic cholangiogram* Stenoses are present in the right and left hepatic ducts. The common hepatic duct is irregular in outline but the cystic duct is normal. No calculi are present

9.3 **Primary sclerosing cholangitis** A 29-year-old male with mild total colitis since the age of 14 who developed jaundice with fevers and steatorrhoea *Endoscopic cholangiogram* The common hepatic and common bile ducts are dilated with an irregular outline; no filling of intrahepatic ducts could be achieved. At laparotomy the common bile duct had a very thick wall, the right hepatic duct was narrowed and the left hepatic duct had barely any lumen. No evidence of carcinoma or calculi was found

9.2

9.3

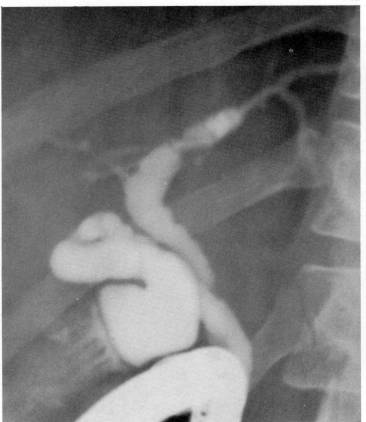

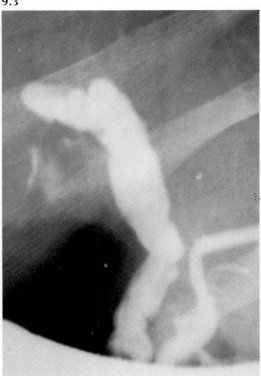

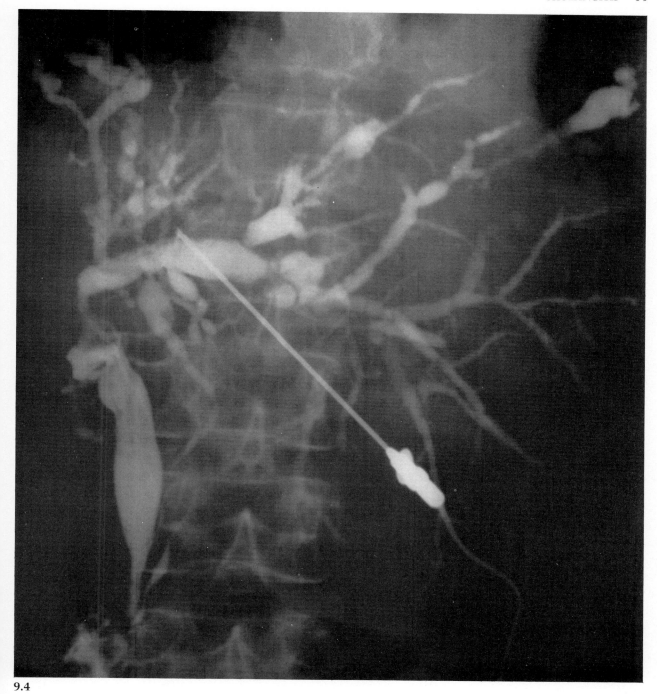

9.4

9.4 Primary sclerosing cholangitis *Percutaneous cholangiogram* Multiple short strictures of the intrahepatic ducts have produced a beaded appearance. The ducts in the right lobe of the liver have not filled and the common hepatic duct and the lower common bile duct are narrowed. Linear filling defects in the dilated upper common bile duct are probably due to inspissated bile (Courtesy of Dr. R.D. Dick)

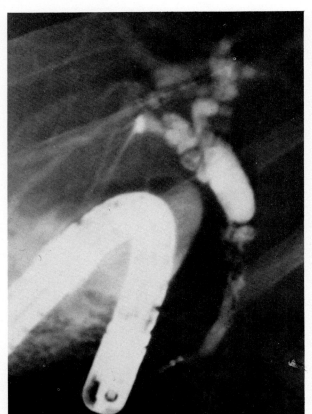

9.5 **Primary sclerosing cholangitis** (Burwood *et al.* 1973) A 37-year-old male with longstanding ulcerative colitis who developed jaundice with bouts of abdominal pain *Endoscopic cholangiogram* Multiple short strictures are apparent in the common bile duct and in the upper common hepatic and intrahepatic ducts. The gallbladder contains many small calculi and several others are present in the common hepatic and bile ducts. At operation the common bile duct was found to be thickened and to contain pigment stones which were also present in the enlarged gallbladder; biopsy confirmed sclerosing cholangitis. Cholecystectomy and choledochoduodenostomy were performed and the patient was quite well three years later

9.6 **Primary biliary cirrhosis** A middle-aged woman with jaundice; mitochondrial antibodies were present and liver biopsy was confirmatory *Endoscopic cholangiogram* a The intrahepatic bile ducts have an irregular calibre and some are tortuous in configuration. b The common hepatic and common bile ducts are normal

9.6b

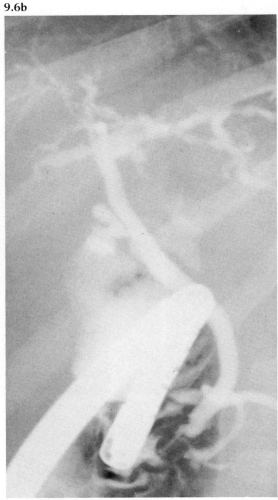

9.5

9.6a

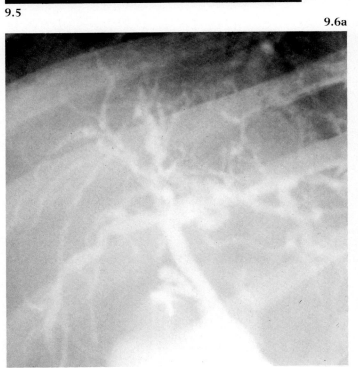

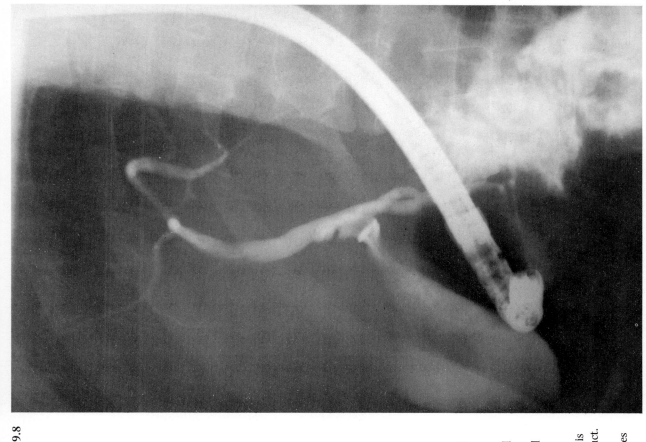

9.8

9.7

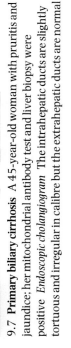

9.7 **Primary biliary cirrhosis** A 45-year-old woman with pruritis and jaundice; her mitochondrial antibody test and liver biopsy were positive *Endoscopic cholangiogram* The intrahepatic ducts are slightly tortuous and irregular in calibre but the extrahepatic ducts are normal

9.8 **Primary biliary cirrhosis with a normal biliary tree** A 32-year-old man with a 7-year history of recurrent upper abdominal pain, and a 6-week history of episodic obstructive jaundice. *Endoscopic retrograde cholangio-pancreatogram* The biliary tree is normal and the gallbladder is filled. Note the course of the cystic duct posterior to the common bile duct. The pancreatogram shows an isolated Wirsung system. Note acinar filling of the ventral pancreas, its downward course and, where it crosses L2 and L3, the impression made by the superior mesenteric artery

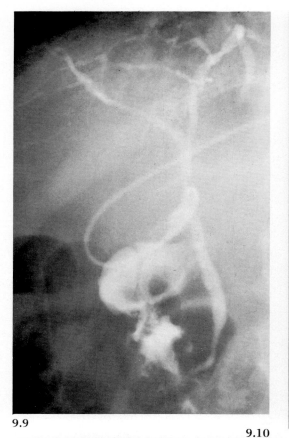

9.9

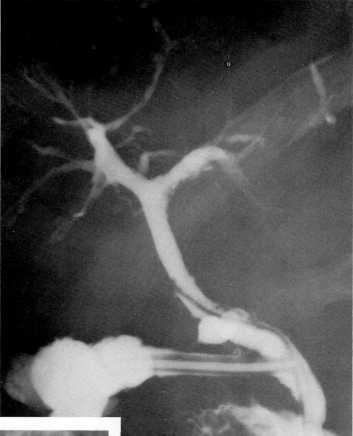

9.10

9.11

9.9 **Mucoviscidosis and hepatic fibrosis**
A seven-year-old child with mucoviscidosis
and jaundice *Operative cholangiogram* The
intrahepatic ducts are irregular in calibre
and hypoplastic but the extrahepatic ducts
are normal. Liver biopsy revealed hepatic
fibrosis of the type found in patients with
mucoviscidosis (Courtesy of Dr. I.R.S.
Gordon)
9.10 **Mucoviscidosis and hepatic fibrosis**
A 16-year-old boy with mucoviscidosis who
became jaundiced *Endoscopic cholangiogram*
The intrahepatic ducts show minor
irregularities in calibre similar to those
seen in primary biliary cirrhosis
9.11 **Sclerosing cholangitis** A young man
with chronic ulcerative colitis *T-tube
cholangiogram* There are short strictures
with marked distortion of the intrahepatic
bile ducts and the left hepatic duct is
irregular. The common hepatic and common
bile ducts have a serrated outline.

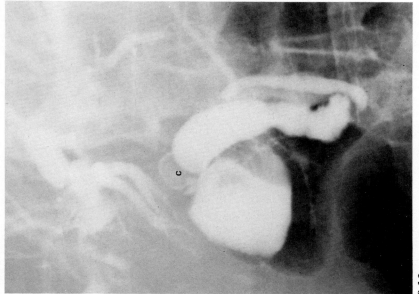

9.13

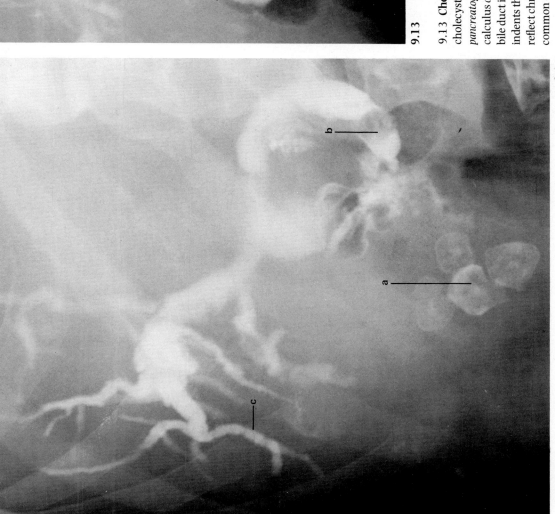

9.12

9.13 Cholangitis secondary to bile duct calculus Previous cholecystectomy *Endoscopic cholangiogram and pancreatogram* The bile ducts are dilated and there is a calculus *c* in the upper common bile duct; the lower common bile duct is irregular in calibre with a serrated outline and indents the pancreatic duct. These radiological appearances reflect chronic inflammatory changes and ulceration of the common duct due to the calculus

9.12 Suppurative cholangitis secondary to biliary calculi An elderly patient who, having tolerated biliary symptoms, developed obstructive jaundice and fever *Endoscopic cholangiogram* There are four opaque calculi in the gallbladder *a*, which has not been outlined by contrast medium because of cystic duct obstruction. A lucent calculus *b* is present in the lower common bile duct, and the intrahepatic bile ducts are dilated and have a serrated outline which gives some of the smaller ducts a beaded appearance *c*

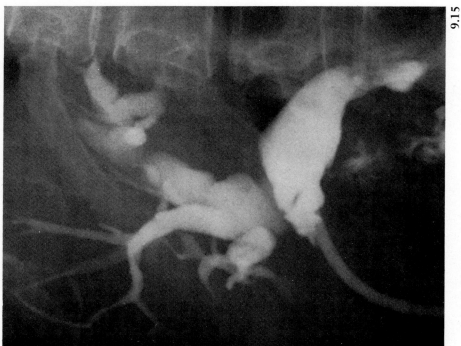

9.14   Suppurative cholangitis secondary to bile duct calculus
Operative cholangiogram The common bile duct is obstructed by a radiolucent calculus at the papilla and no contrast medium has entered the duodenum. The bile ducts are dilated and the intrahepatic ducts are irregular in calibre and show a serrated outline

9.15   Recurrent pyogenic cholangitis—Oriental cholangitis
(Wastie & Cunningham 1973) A 58-year-old Chinese woman from Malaysia; there was no evidence of Clonorchis infestation *T-tube cholangiogram* The common duct is dilated and there are strictures and dilatation of the hepatic ducts, but the right duct is much less affected; this is a feature of oriental cholangitis

9.15

9.14

9.17

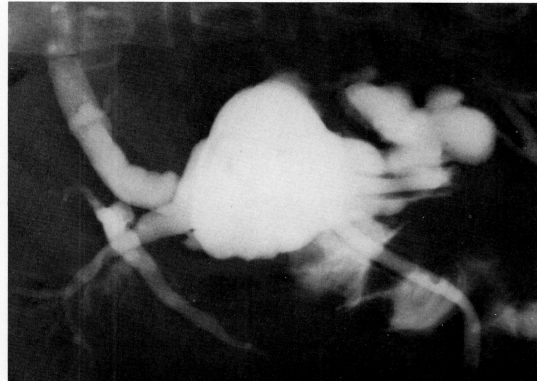

9.16

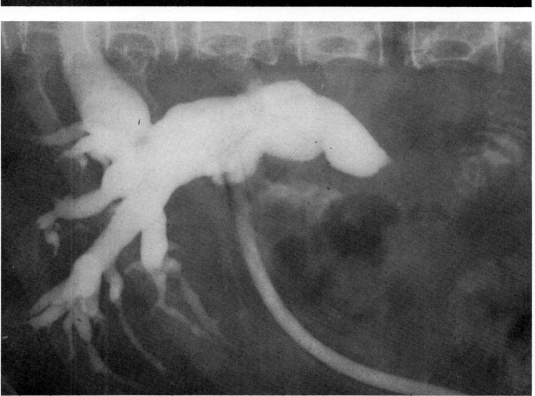

9.16 **Recurrent pyogenic cholangitis** (Wastie & Cunningham 1973) A 52-year-old Chinese woman from Malaysia *T-tube cholangiogram* The bile ducts are dilated, but there are major strictures of the intrahepatic ducts in the right lobe

9.17 **Recurrent pyogenic cholangitis** (Wastie & Cunningham 1973) A 19-year-old Chinese girl from Malaysia *T-tube cholangiogram* There are multiple strictures in the dilated common bile duct with a marked stricture at its lower end. Reflux into the pancreatic duct has occurred. The left hepatic duct is more dilated than the right

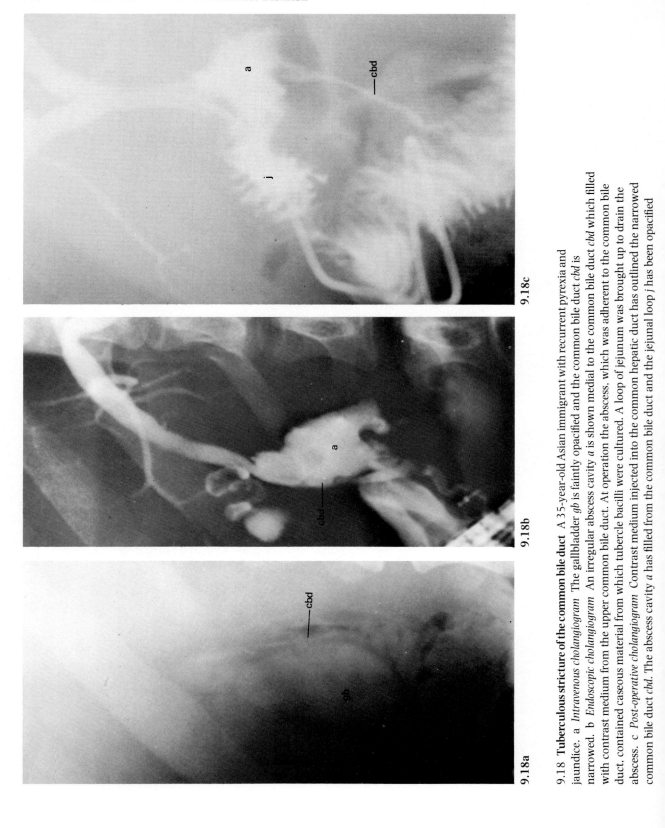

9.18 **Tuberculous stricture of the common bile duct** A 35-year-old Asian immigrant with recurrent pyrexia and jaundice. a *Intravenous cholangiogram* The gallbladder *gb* is faintly opacified and the common bile duct *cbd* is narrowed. b *Endoscopic cholangiogram* An irregular abscess cavity *a* is shown medial to the common bile duct *cbd* which filled with contrast medium from the upper common bile duct. At operation the abscess, which was adherent to the common bile duct, contained caseous material from which tubercle bacilli were cultured. A loop of jejunum was brought up to drain the abscess. c *Post-operative cholangiogram* Contrast medium injected into the common hepatic duct has outlined the narrowed common bile duct *cbd*. The abscess cavity *a* has filled from the common bile duct and the jejunal loop *j* has been opacified

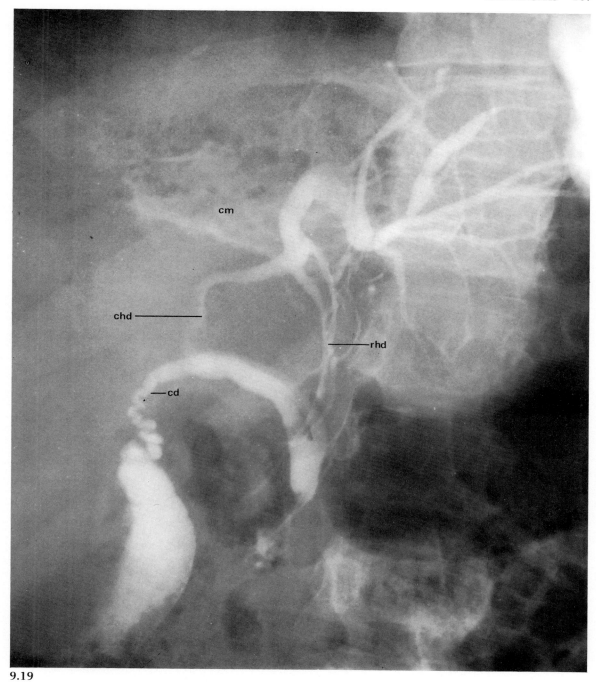

9.19

9.19 Hydatid cyst in right lobe of the liver *Endoscopic cholangiogram* There is a large space-occupying lesion in the right lobe which is displacing and compressing the common hepatic duct *chd*. The right hepatic ducts *rhd* are displaced towards the midline. The cystic duct *cd* overlies the common hepatic duct *chd* and they unite low down behind the pancreas. Contrast medium *cm* has extravasated from the bile ducts into the space surrounding the hydatid cyst

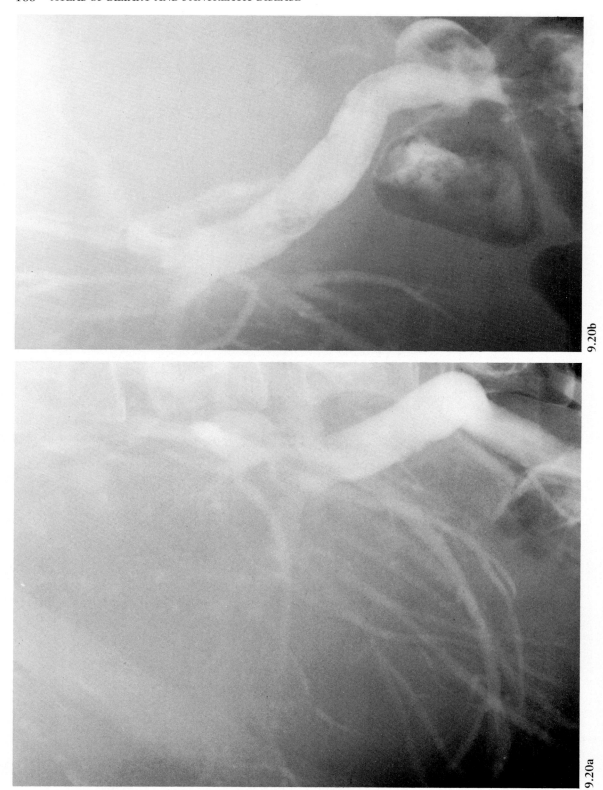

9.20a

9.20b

9.20 **Hydatid cyst in the right lobe of liver** *Endoscopic cholangiogram* a The intrahepatic ducts in the right lobe are displaced downward and medially by the space occupying lesion. b Band-like filling defects in the common hepatic and common bile ducts proved at operation to be due to the wall of a ruptured hydatid cyst

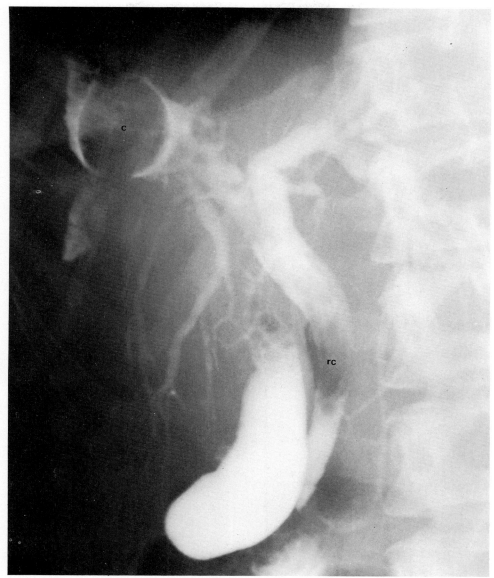

9.21

9.21 Recurrent hydatid cyst A 23-year-old woman after removal of a hydatid cyst from the right lobe of the liver. The intrahepatic tube continued to drain bile and a sinogram showed a daughter cyst within the cavity of the previous cyst. Retrograde cholangiography was performed to demonstrate the bile ducts *Endoscopic cholangiogram* An oval filling defect *rc* seen in the common bile duct was found at operation to be due to a ruptured hydatid cyst. The daughter cyst *c* is shown as a round filling defect within the cavity of the previous cyst which has been outlined by contrast medium. Two smaller cysts are present above it

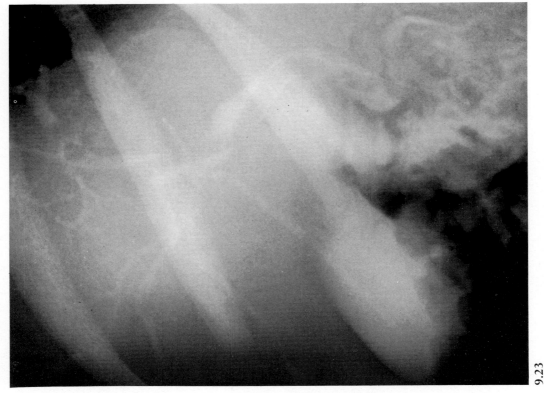

9.23

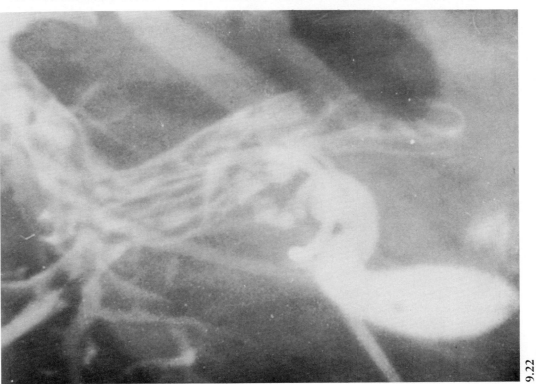

9.22

9.22 **Roundworms in the bile ducts** *Operative cholangiogram* Numerous band-like filling defects caused by the presence of roundworms can be seen within the dilated right and left common hepatic ducts. One worm has entered the gallbladder (Courtesy of Dr. Kyaw Aung)

9.23 **Roundworm in the bile ducts** *Intravenous cholangiogram* There is a linear filling defect in the common hepatic and common bile ducts (Courtesy of Prof. B.J. Cremin & Dr. D.J. Mackenzie-Crooks)

10 Biliary Fistula

Spontaneous biliary enteric fistulae are most often caused by calculi eroding the walls of the biliary tract and entering an adjacent hollow viscus. Chronic calculus cholecystitis with fistula to either the duodenum or colon is the commonest aetiology. Calculi in the lower common bile duct may erode its wall and form a biliary-enteric fistula adjacent to the duodenal papilla. Benign peptic ulcers of the stomach or duodenum may erode the common bile duct and carcinomas in the gallbladder or bowel may erode into an adjacent hollow viscus. The number of fistulae due to Crohn's disease of the bowel is increasing (Safaie-Shirazi *et al.* 1973). Inflammatory lesions in the liver may lead to fistulae between the biliary tree and the pleural cavity. Amoebic or purulent liver abscesses and hydatid disease may be responsible. Gallstones have been recorded as ulcerating through the diaphragm into the lung (Schwegler & Endrei 1975).

Although biliary enteric fistulae are now relatively rare and are discovered about once in every hundred cholecystectomies, they were once common; the diminished incidence is due to modern biliary surgery for cholelithiasis. Small biliary fistulae may be found incidentally at cholecystectomy for cholecystitis, but more often they are associated with febrile episodes due to contamination of the bile ducts with gut bacteria. Colonic fistulae may produce so much contamination that bile salts become deconjugated and steatorrhoea may develop (Gudas *et al.* 1967). Ulceration of a large calculus from the biliary tree into the small bowel may produce acute gallstone obstruction of the small bowel as well as a biliary fistula. Such calculi usually traverse the small bowel to impact in the terminal ileum, which is of smaller calibre than the jejunum.

Biliary enteric fistulae are characterized by the presence of gas in the intrahepatic bile ducts which is evident on plain abdominal radiographs. Intravenous cholangiography has been said to be unrewarding, but the method can still be of value in recognizing the fistulous viscus. If there is plain film evidence of small bowel obstruction a diagnosis of gallstone obstruction can be suggested, especially so if the offending stone is calcified and can be recognized on the film. Barium studies of the upper gastrointestinal tract may reveal fistulae due to peptic ulceration and barium enema examination may demonstrate a cholecystocolic fistula. Endoscopic cholangiography has proved helpful in the small number of patients so far examined by this technique; small fistulae adjacent to the papilla may be recognized during duodenoscopic cannulation.

References

Safaie-Shirazi S., Zike W. L. & Printen K. J. (1973) *Surg. Gynec. Obstet.*, **137**, 769

Schwegler N. & Endrei E. (1975) *Radiology*, **115**, 541

Gudas P. P., Haberman G. C. & Belcher H. V. (1967) *Arch. Surg.*, **95**, 228

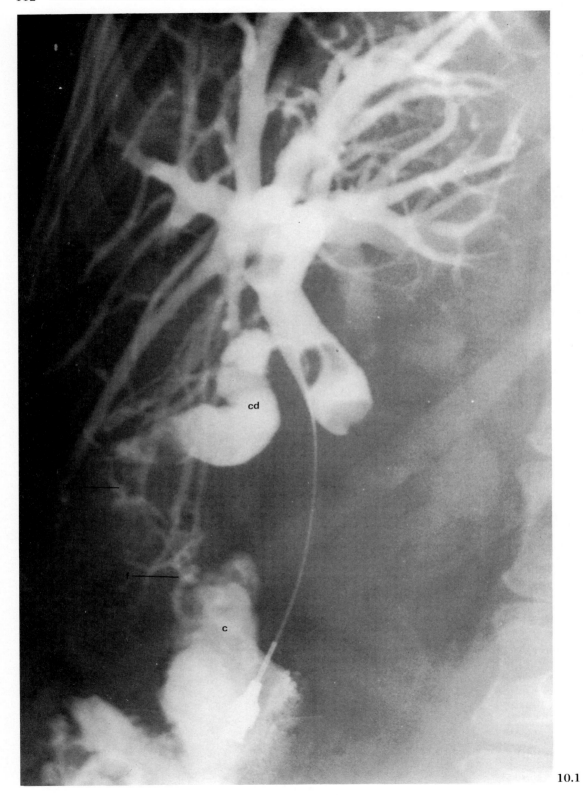

10.1

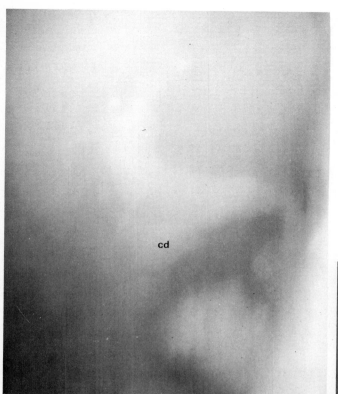

10.2a

only a short segment of dilated cystic duct *cd* has opacified. A diagnosis of cystic duct obstruction was made, but operation was refused. Eighteen months later the patient presented with a fluctuant mass in the right side of the abdomen which discharged pus through a sinus on to the anterior abdominal wall.
b *Sinogram* Contrast medium injected through the catheter has filled the irregular fistulous track *f* and outlined the gallbladder, which contains a radiolucent calculus *c*

10.2b

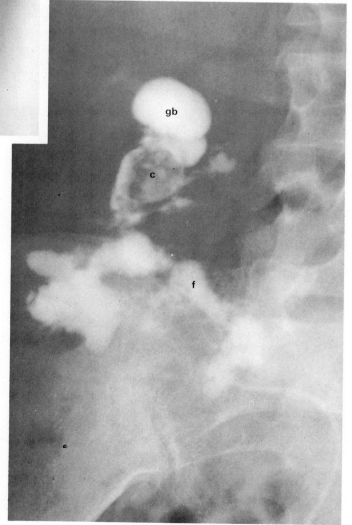

Opposite page
10.1 **Cholecysto-colic fistula complicating cholelithiasis and chronic cholecystitis** A 41-year-old woman with a one-month history of malaise and jaundice. The initial diagnosis was infective hepatitis but liver biopsy suggested extrahepatic duct obstruction *Percutaneous cholangiogram* The intrahepatic ducts are dilated and the common bile duct is obstructed by calculi. Although the cystic duct *cd* is dilated, the gallbladder *gb* is strictured, contracted and contains several calculi. Contrast medium has passed from the fundus of the gallbladder through the fistula *f* into the colon *c*. At laparotomy the fibrotic contracted gallbladder was adherent to the hepatic flexure, and the presence of a cholecysto-colic fistula, gallbladder and bile duct calculi were confirmed (Courtesy of Dr. G. Evison)

10.2 **Biliary fistula complicating chronic cholecystitis and gallbladder calculi** A 56-year-old woman with symptoms of chronic cholecystitis showed no opacification of the gallbladder at oral cholecystography. a *Intravenous cholangiography and tomography* The common duct is dilated and has no calculi within it. The gallbladder is not outlined and

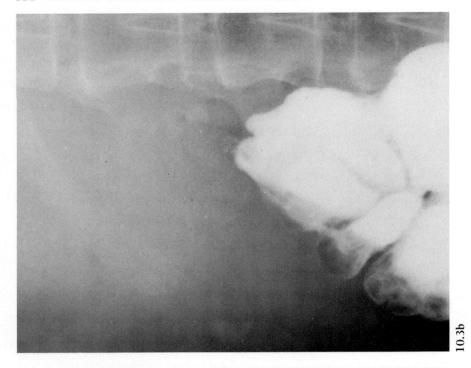

10.3b

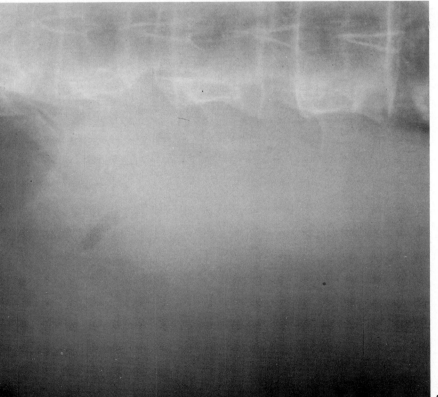

10.3a

10.3 **Cholecysto-colic fistula complicating chronic cholecystitis** A 54-year-old man presented with steatorrhoea and weight loss; he also complained of febrile episodes and was mildly jaundiced. Small bowel barium meal examination was initially reported as normal, but at laparotomy a scarred and contracted gallbladder was found adherent to the hepatic flexure and a fistula was demonstrated. a *Preliminary plain abdomen film of small bowel examination* A short linear gas lucency overlies the upper liver, consistent with a small amount of gas in the biliary tree. b *Late film of small bowel barium examination* Barium has entered the hepatic flexure of the colon and a small amount has passed upwards to the right of the body of L1 in the gallbladder area. A gas lucency overlies the last rib

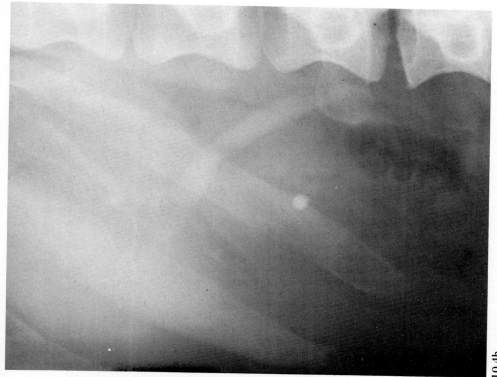

10.4a

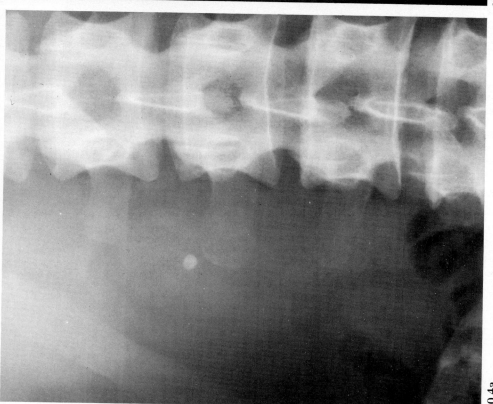

10.4b

10.4 **Gallstone obstruction of the small bowel** A 52-year-old man with symptoms suggestive of gallbladder disease. a *Plain abdomen film* A faint round opacity 4 cm in diameter surrounds a small dense opacity which lies above the right transverse process of L3. b *Intravenous cholangiogram* The common duct is normal in calibre, but there is no opacification of the gallbladder because it is occupied by a large, faintly opaque calculus with a small dense nucleus. Three months after this investigation and whilst awaiting elective cholecystectomy the patient developed acute intestinal obstruction (*continued overleaf*)

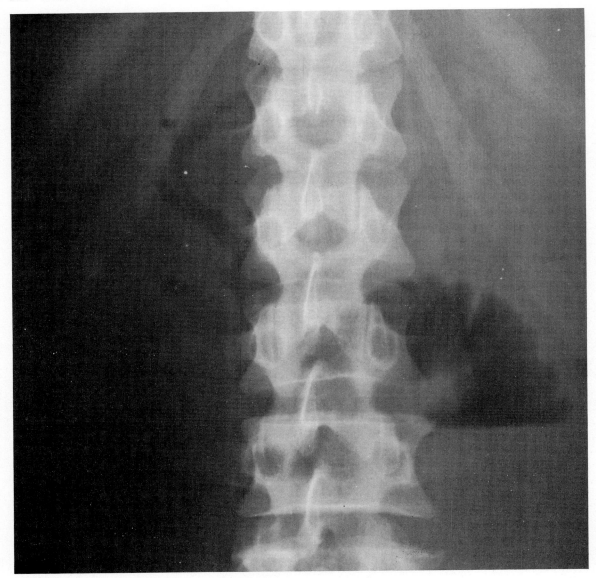

10.4c

10.4 c *Erect abdomen film—three months later* The previous opacity in the gallbladder area is no longer visible but there is gas in the biliary tree and a gas-distended loop of small bowel with a gas/liquid level is evident to the left of the spine. At operation a large gallstone was found to be obstructing the lower ileum and there was a fistula between the gallbladder and the duodenum through which the calculus had passed into the gut (Courtesy of Dr. J. Roylance)

Opposite page

10.5 **Gallstone obstruction of the small bowel** *Supine abdomen film* There is air *a* in the biliary tree and gallbladder owing to a cholecysto-duodenal fistula, and marked gaseous distention of small bowel loops *b* is evident. An opaque calculus *c* is impacted in the distal ileum; the opacity over the sacrum is a calcified lymph node

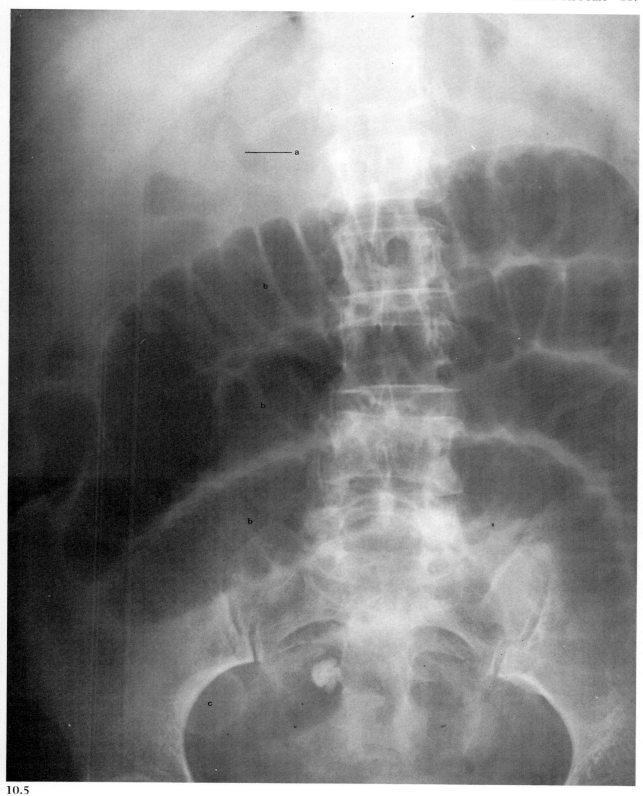

10.5

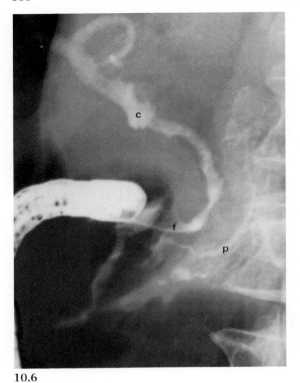

10.6

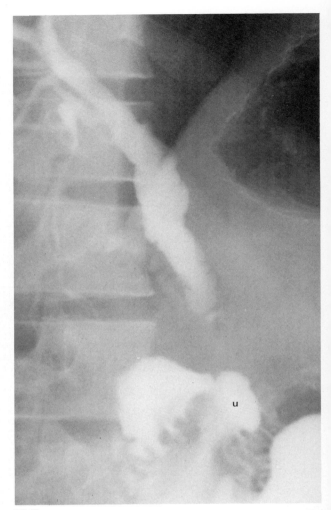

10.7a

10.7b

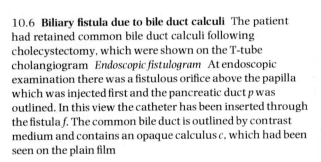

10.6 Biliary fistula due to bile duct calculi The patient had retained common bile duct calculi following cholecystectomy, which were shown on the T-tube cholangiogram *Endoscopic fistulogram* At endoscopic examination there was a fistulous orifice above the papilla which was injected first and the pancreatic duct *p* was outlined. In this view the catheter has been inserted through the fistula *f*. The common bile duct is outlined by contrast medium and contains an opaque calculus *c*, which had been seen on the plain film

10.7 Biliary fistula due to duodenal ulceration A 35-year-old West African with dyspepsia *Barium meal examination* a The duodenal bulb has been replaced by a giant peptic duodenal ulcer crater *u*; the pyloric antrum is indented by the oedematous rim of the crater and barium is present within the common bile duct. b An oblique view shows the fistula between the posterior aspect of the giant crater and the common bile duct

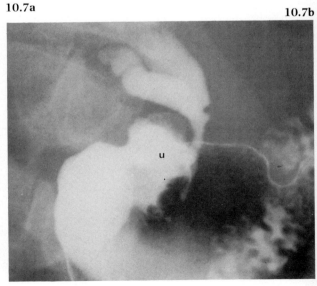

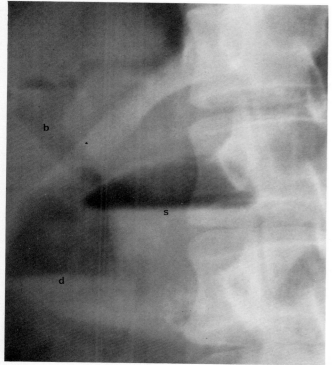

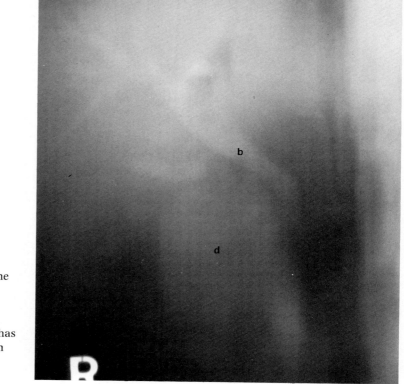

**10.8 Choledocho-duodenal fistula due to
Crohn's disease** A 27-year-old man with
vomiting and loss of weight.   a *Erect plain
abdomen film* There is gas in the biliary tree *b*.
Gas/liquid levels are present in the antrum of the
stomach *s* and descending duodenum *d*.
b *Intravenous cholangiogram with tomography*
Despite the presence of gas in the bile ducts, a
good visualization of the common bile duct *b* has
been obtained. Contrast medium has pooled in
the distended descending duodenum *d*
(continued overleaf)

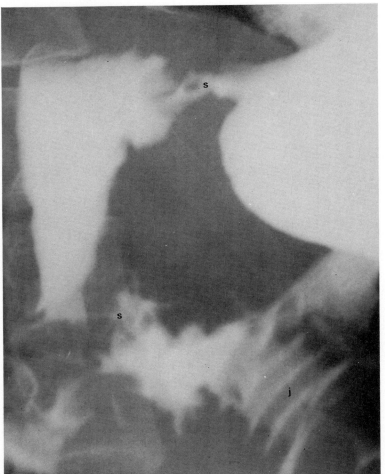

10.8c

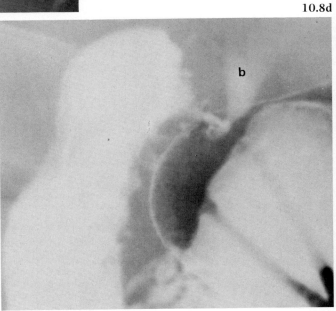

10.8d

Opposite page

10.9 **Choledocho-duodenal fistula due to Crohn's disease** A young man with pyloric obstruction caused by Crohn's disease of the duodenum and pylorus. a *Endoscopic cannulation of the small bowel* A catheter has been advanced through the strictured pylorus under direct endoscopic inspection to outline the irregular stricture of the duodenum and pylorus. The stomach is grossly distended and the gastric antrum lies to the right of the duodenum; there is gas in the biliary tree. b *Endoscopic cannulation of the biliary tree* At a second investigation a catheter passed from the first part of the duodenum through a fistula into the biliary tree. The contrast medium filled gallbladder overlies the catheter (*continued*)

10.8 c *Barium meal examination* There is irregular narrowing *s* of the first part and lower descending duodenum, and the duodenum lying between is distended; a deformed jejunal loop *j* with thickened folds overlies the third part. The appearances are those of Crohn's disease involving the duodenum and jejunum. d *Barium meal examination* A coned view of the strictured first part of duodenum reveals the fistula between the involved duodenal bulb and the lower common bile duct *b*

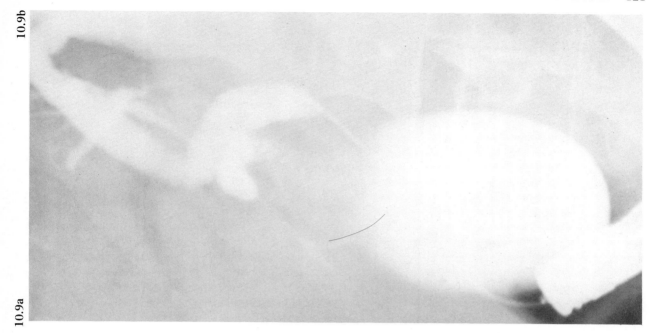

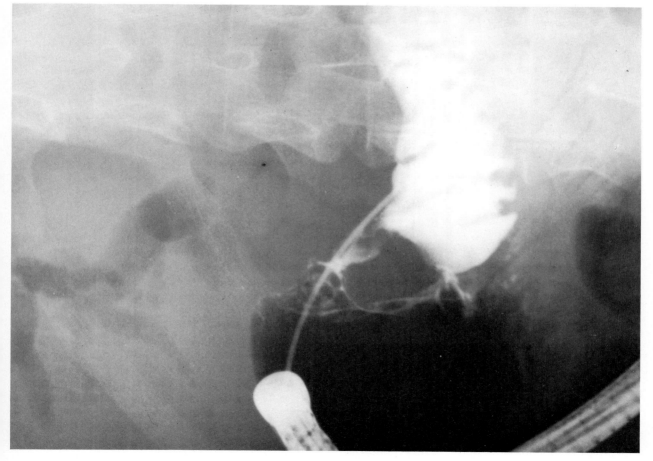

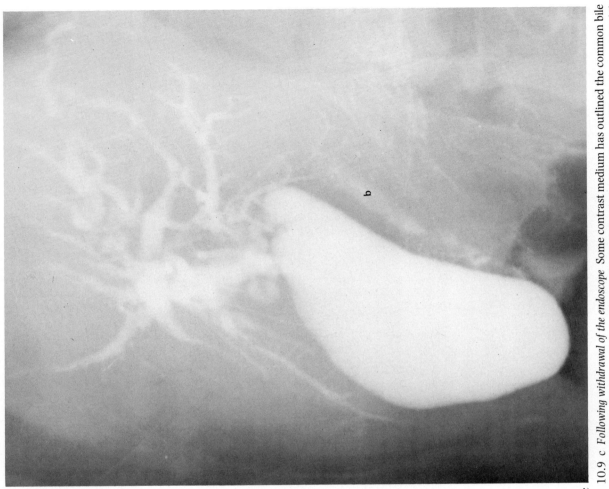

10.9c

10.9 c *Following withdrawal of the endoscope* Some contrast medium has outlined the common bile duct *b* below the fistula and adjacent to the diseased descending duodenum. The lower common bile duct shows irregular narrowing caused by Crohn's disease

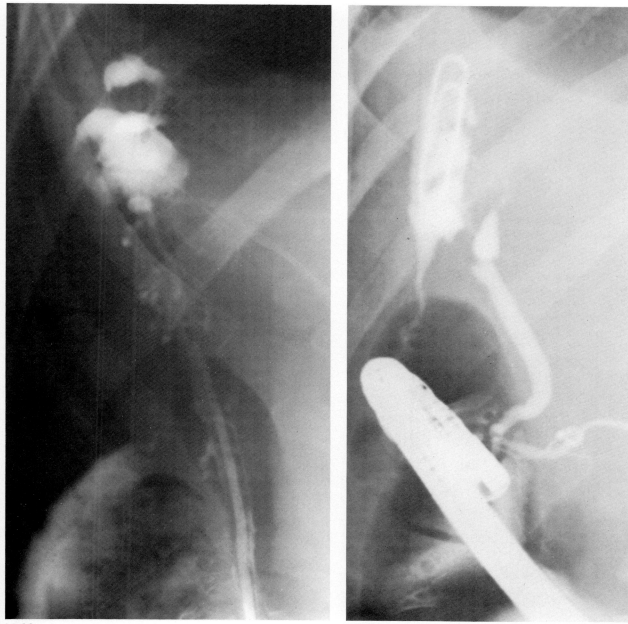

10.10a

10.10b

10.10 **Biliary fistula following laceration of the liver** A 21-year-old woman had a right lobectomy following severe laceration of the liver in a road traffic accident; there was a persistent bile leak from the tube drain. a *Sinogram* An irregular sinus cavity is outlined in the liver bed. b *Endoscopic cholangiogram* There is a small fistula between the left hepatic duct and the cavity outlined at sinography. A paper-clip on the skin overlies the cavity

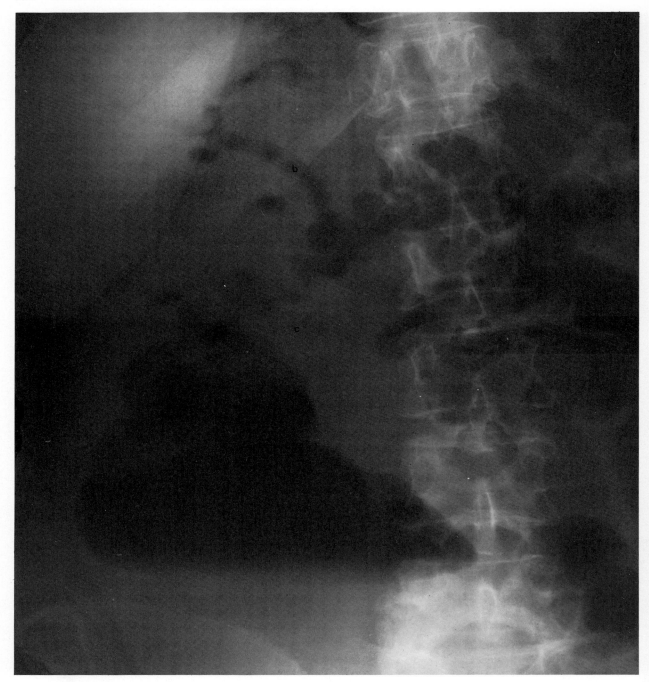

10.11 Cholecystocolic fistula due to carcinoma of the hepatic flexure An elderly woman with intestinal obstruction and cholangitis *Erect plain abdomen film* A lobulated filling defect due to carcinoma *c* is outlined by gas in the hepatic flexure. Gas is present in the biliary tree *b*, and the caecum is distended and contains a long gas/liquid level; distended small bowel loops are present to the left of the spine. At laparotomy a carcinoma was found to be obstructing the hepatic flexure and invading the gallbladder

Tumours of the gallbladder

Benign polyps Benign polypoid tumours may be demonstrated as radiolucent filling defects within the gallbladder at oral cholecystography. They differ from calculi in that they maintain their position within the gallbladder in different projections and are usually less than 1 cm in diameter; profile views may show their attachment to the wall of the gallbladder. The majority of polypoid lesions are cholesterol or adenomyomatous polyps which have already been considered in Chapter 7. Only 4 per cent. of such tumours are true adenomata, and follow up of polypoid lesions of the gallbladder, diagnosed by oral cholecystography, failed to show evidence of developing carcinoma (Selzer *et al.* 1962).

Primary gallbladder carcinoma Although often considered to be uncommon, primary gallbladder carcinoma has been shown to account for about 1 per cent. of all carcinomas in Great Britain (Cooke *et al.* 1953) and occurs most often in women in whom there is a high incidence of concomitant cholecystitis and cholelithiasis; coexistent calculi are found less frequently in men with the disease. Adenocarcinoma is the most common histological type. Patients may present with symptoms of acute or chronic cholecystitis or with jaundice and loss of weight, but there may be no history of previous gallbladder disease.

Opacification of the gallbladder was not achieved by either oral cholecystography or intravenous cholangiography in any of 27 patients studied by Donaldson & Busuttil (1975) although opaque calculi were seen on the preliminary film in three instances. Percutaneous or endoscopic cholangiography may show stricture or obstruction of the common hepatic or common bile ducts.

Most tumours involve the right lobe of the liver or adjacent hollow viscera at the time of presentation and the prognosis for patients with unresectable tumours is poor (*Lancet* 1971). Because of the implied risk of carcinoma in patients with gallbladder stones, prophylactic cholecystectomy has been advocated for all patients with radiological evidence of calculi (Prakash *et al.* 1975).

References

Cooke L., Avery-Jones F. & Keech M.K. (1953) *Lancet*, **ii**, 585

Donaldson L.A. & Busuttil A. (1975) *Brit. J. Surg.*, **62**, 26

Leading article (1971) *Lancet*, **ii**, 967

Prakash A.T.M., Sharma L.K. & Pandit P.N. (1975) *Brit. J. Surg.*, **62**, 33

Selzer D.W., Dockerty M.B., Stauffer M.H. & Priestley J.T. (1962) *Amer. J. Surg.*, **103**, 472

Tumours of the bile ducts

Benign tumours of the bile ducts presenting with symptoms are extremely rare and they usually remain undetected until there is evidence of biliary obstruction and cholangitis (Dowdy *et al.* 1962). Papillomatous lesions can be single or multiple and may have malignant potential. Adenomata may grow to a large size before presentation.

11 Neoplastic Disease of the Biliary Tract

Bile duct carcinoma Although less common than carcinoma of the pancreas or gallbladder, bile duct carcinoma is quite a frequent cause of bile duct obstruction. The lesions are usually adenocarcinomas which may involve the right and left intrahepatic ducts as often as the common hepatic duct, and there is an increased incidence in patients with ulcerative colitis (Roberts-Thomson *et al.* 1973) and Caroli's disease (Gallagher *et al.* 1972). Patients are usually over 50 years of age and present with progressive obstructive jaundice and weight loss. Carcinoma of the pancreas or periampullary region is commonly suspected but the gallbladder cannot be palpated.

Endoscopic cholangiography is the best method of investigation for demonstrating the level of obstruction and should be attempted first, but if endoscopic cholangiography proves impossible or if total obstruction is shown at retrograde examination, percutaneous cholangiography can then be used to demonstrate the upper limit of the lesion and the proximal bile ducts. The affected duct may show a shouldered stenosis with a rat-tail configuration or the lesion may produce a polypoid filling defect. The major differentiation is from benign stricture in patients who have had previous biliary surgery. Benign strictures tend to be short and smooth whereas carcinomatous strictures are elongated and associated with filling defects.

Sclerosing cholangitis may also develop in patients with ulcerative colitis and it may be hard to decide whether biliary strictures are due to this cause or to sclerosing cholangiocarcinoma; indeed, the lesions may coexist. Histological examination or follow-up may be necessary to make the differentiation (Altemeier *et al.* 1966).

Hepatic and pancreatic scintigraphy have been advocated for patients with suspected biliary or pancreatic neoplasms (Agnew *et al.* 1975), as there may be areas of impaired uptake of radionuclide adjacent to the hilum because of dilated bile ducts. Ultrasound examination may also demonstrate dilated intrahepatic bile ducts or enlargement of the gallbladder due to lesions involving the lower common bile duct. Surgical resection is seldom possible, and in the majority of cases the surgeon has to be satisfied with some form of palliative procedure.

Extrinsic compression of the common hepatic duct by malignant lymph nodes at the porta hepatis Lymph node metastasis from alimentary tract, lung or breast carcinoma may produce compression and invasion of the common hepatic duct at the portal fissure. This is usually an event in the deterioration of a patient with a known primary neoplasm, although jaundice may be the presenting symptom in some cases. Intrahepatic metastasis may also cause bile duct occlusion. Lymphoma is an uncommon cause of extrahepatic duct obstruction and jaundice is more often due to hepatic parenchymal involvement.

References

Agnew J. E., James O. & Bouchier I. A. D. (1975) *Brit. J. Radiol.*, **48**, 190

Altemeier W. A., Gall E. A., Culbertson W. R. & Inge W. W. (1966) *Surgery*, **60**, 191

Dowdy G. S., Olin W. G., Shelton E. L. & Waldron G. W. (1962) *Arch. Surg.*, **85**, 503

Gallagher P. J., Mills R. R. & Mitchinson M. J. (1972) *J. clin. Path.*, **25**, 804

Roberts-Thomson I. C., Strickland R. G. & Mackay I. R. (1973) *Aust. N.Z. J. Med.*, **3**, 264

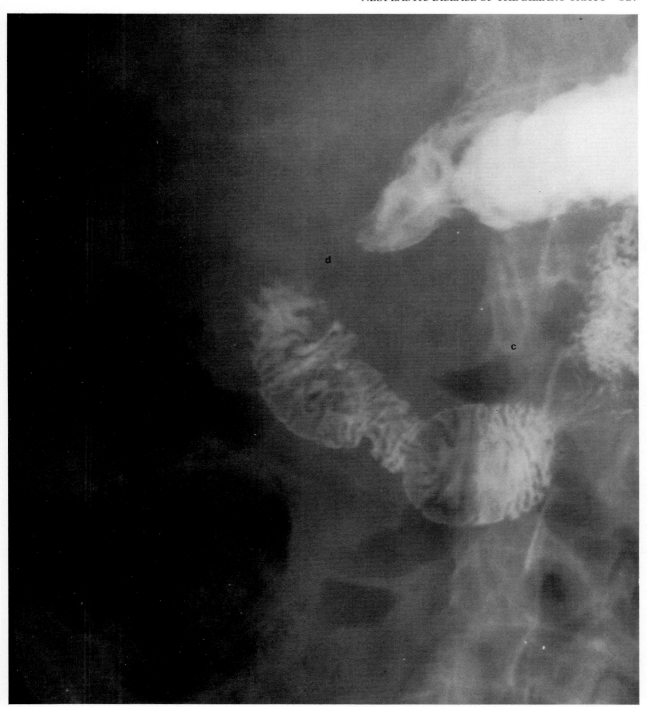

11.1

11.1 **Carcinoma of the gallbladder** An elderly man who complained of abdominal pain and loss of weight. There was a hard mass in the right upper abdomen *Barium meal* There is a stricture of the duodenum *d* due to carcinomatous invasion and the mass is outlined by gas in the colon *c*

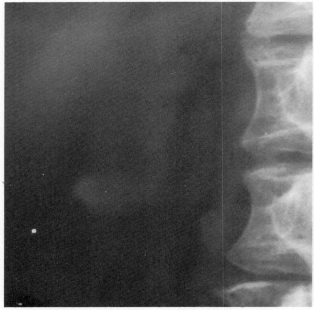

11.2a

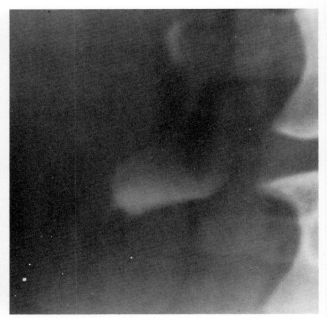

11.2b

11.3

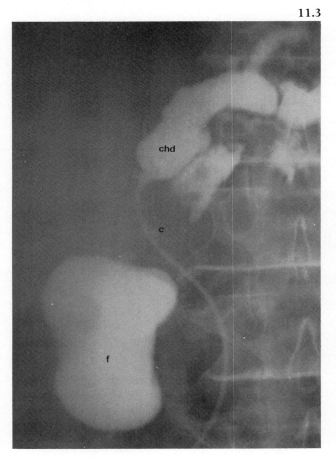

11.2 Carcinoma of the gallbladder A 65-year-old man who presented with ascites and weight loss. There was a palpable mass in the right hypochondrium. Gallbladder carcinoma with widespread peritoneal metastasis was found at laparotomy *Oral cholecystogram* a There is a filling defect in the fundus of the gallbladder and only the upper part of the body has been outlined by contrast medium. b *Coned view*—the upper margin of the tumour is outlined by contrast medium and shows a rat-tail configuration

11.3 Carcinoma of the gallbladder *Operative cholecystogram and cholangiogram* Contrast medium has been injected both into the fundus of gallbladder *f* and into the common hepatic duct *chd* via the catheter. The left hepatic duct is dilated and the right hepatic and common bile ducts and the body of the gallbladder *c* are not opacified. There was a large carcinoma involving the body and neck of the gallbladder which had invaded the common hepatic duct, the common bile duct and the liver

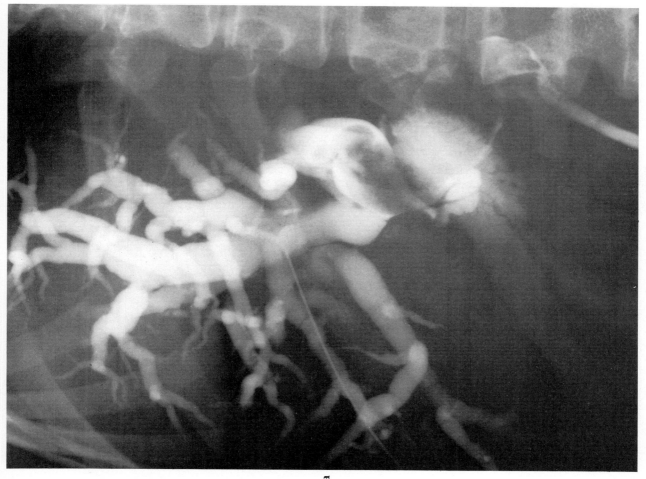

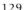

11.5a

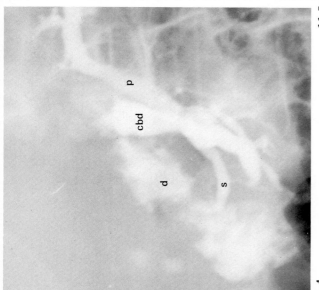

11.4

11.4 Carcinoma of the gallbladder invading the common bile duct A 58-year-old woman with jaundice *Retrograde cholangiogram and pancreatogram* There is occlusion of the common bile duct *cbd* at the level of the upper border of the pancreas. The pancreatic duct *p* is dilated and some contrast medium has drained via the Santorini ducts into the duodenum *d*. At operation the bile duct occlusion was shown to be due to a carcinoma of the gallbladder. There were two opaque calculi in the gallbladder and the pancreas was thickened due to chronic pancreatitis

11.5 Benign papillary adenoma of the common hepatic duct A 52-year-old woman with progressive jaundice.
a *Percutaneous cholangiogram* There is a large polypoid filling defect in the common hepatic and upper common bile duct. The upper margin of the tumour is outlined by contrast medium in the dilated right and left hepatic ducts. Some contrast medium has entered the gallbladder which overlies the lesion and the normal calibre common bile duct below the lesion *(continued overleaf)*

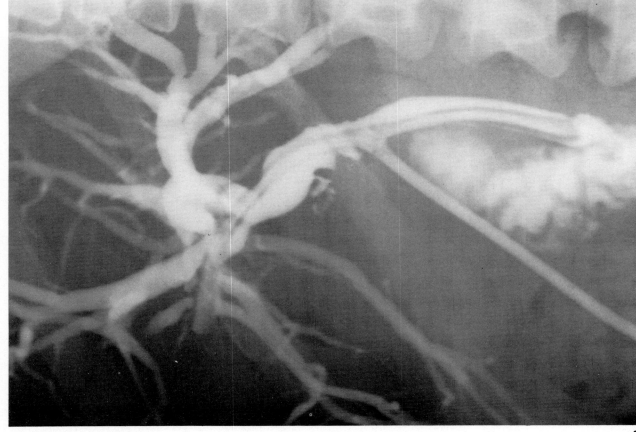

11.5b

11.5 b *T-tube cholangiogram* The tumour has been removed, so that the intrahepatic and common hepatic ducts are less dilated and draining normally (Courtesy of Dr. J. Beales & Dr. G. Evison)

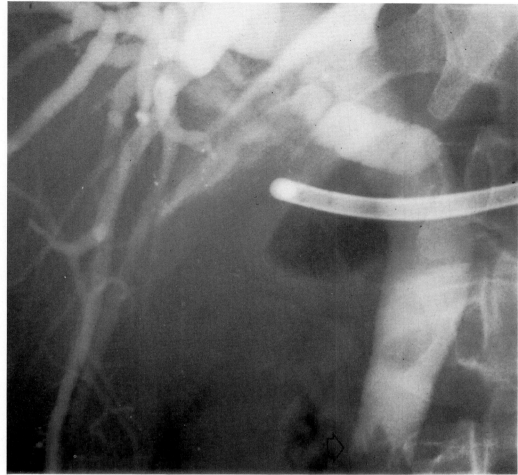

11.6a

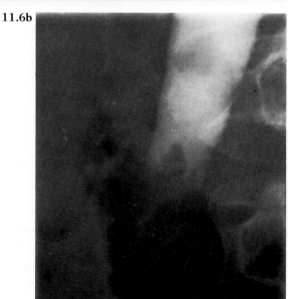

11.6b

11.6 **Benign papilloma of the common bile duct** *Fine-needle cholangiography* a A filling defect with an irregular upper margin is seen obstructing the common bile duct. b Coned view of the papilloma (Courtesy of Dr. D.J. Lintott)

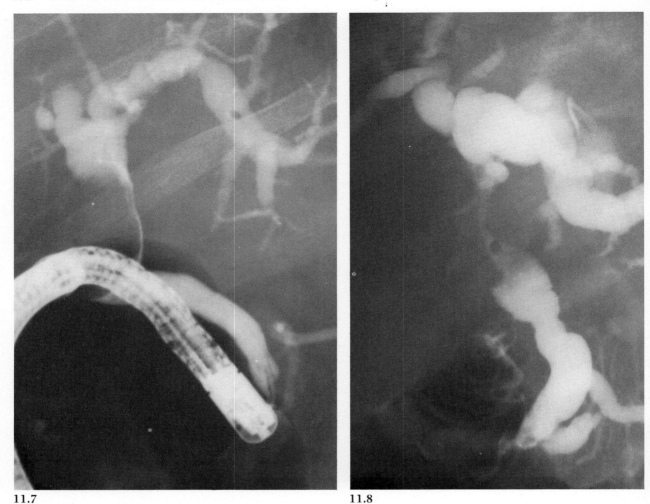

11.7

11.8

11.7 Polypoid carcinoma of the common hepatic duct A 60-year-old man with jaundice *Endoscopic cholangiogram* There is a well-defined oval filling defect in the common hepatic duct which was found at operation to be due to a poorly differentiated adenocarcinoma.

11.8 Annular carcinoma of the common hepatic duct A 63-year-old woman with jaundice *Endoscopic cholangiogram* There is a 4-cm-long irregular stricture of the common hepatic duct with dilatation of the intrahepatic ducts. The cystic duct and gallbladder have not filled

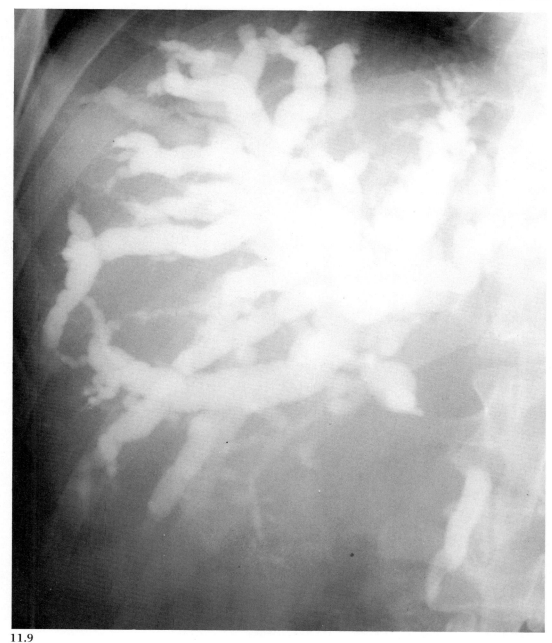

11.9

11.9 Tapering stricture of the common hepatic duct due to cholangiocarcinoma *Percutaneous cholangiogram* The intrahepatic ducts and a short segment of common duct are dilated above the tapered occlusion. Some contrast medium has passed into the lower common bile duct

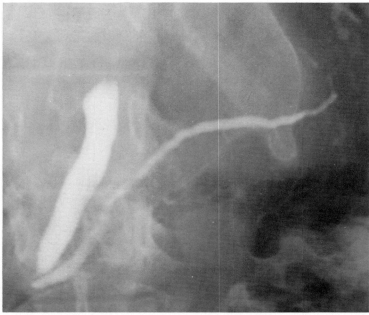

11.10

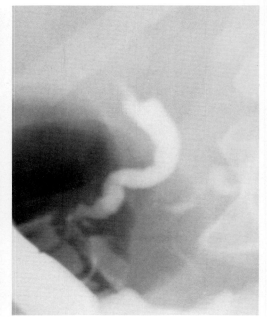

11.11

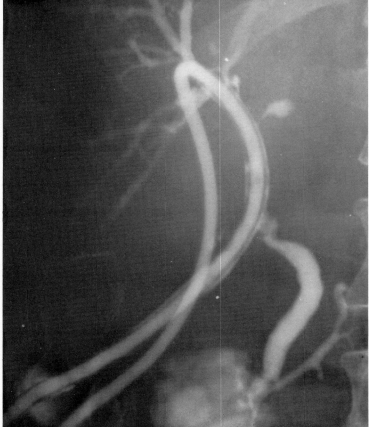

11.12

11.10 **Occlusion of common bile duct by cholangiocarcinoma** *Endoscopic retrograde cholangiogram and pancreatogram* There is an abrupt occlusion of the common bile duct due to the tumour. The pancreatic duct is normal in calibre

11.11 **Occlusion of the common bile duct by cholangiocarcinoma** *Endoscopic cholangiogram* In addition to occlusion of the common bile duct the lower margins of the lesion show as shouldered filling defects on either side of the narrowed channel

11.12 **Common hepatic duct carcinoma** *U-tube cholangiogram* A U-tube has been inserted through the malignant stricture from below and passed through the surface of the liver and skin. The tube has side holes to aid the drainage of bile from above the neoplasm. Some contrast medium has refluxed into the pancreatic duct.

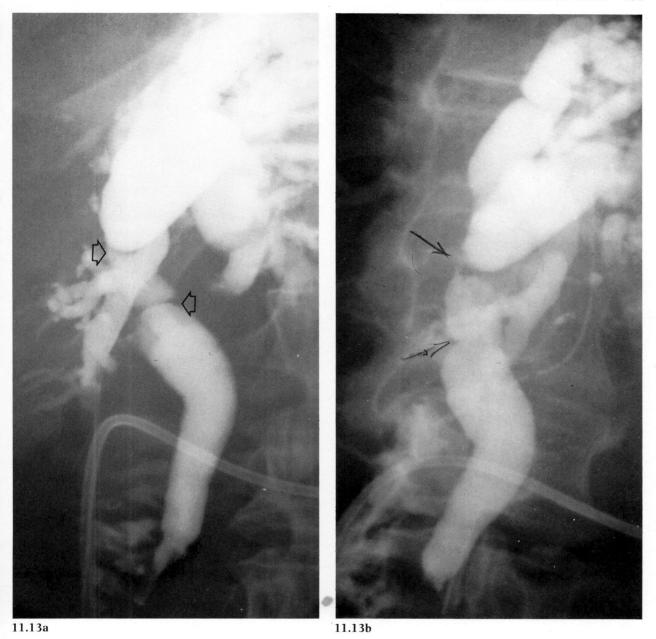

11.13a   **11.13b**

11.13 **Coexistent traumatic and neoplastic strictures of the common hepatic duct** An elderly man who had undergone cholecystectomy several years previously developed progressive jaundice. Coexistent traumatic and adenocarcinomatous strictures were found at operation *Percutaneous cholangiogram* a The common hepatic duct is markedly dilated above the level of the carcinoma (upper arrow) and the short traumatic stricture, 2 cm below it, is well outlined (lower arrow). b On the oblique view the carcinomatous stricture (upper arrow) is 1 cm long and has shouldered margins, whereas the traumatic stricture (lower arrow) is much shorter (Courtesy of Dr. T.A.S. Buist)

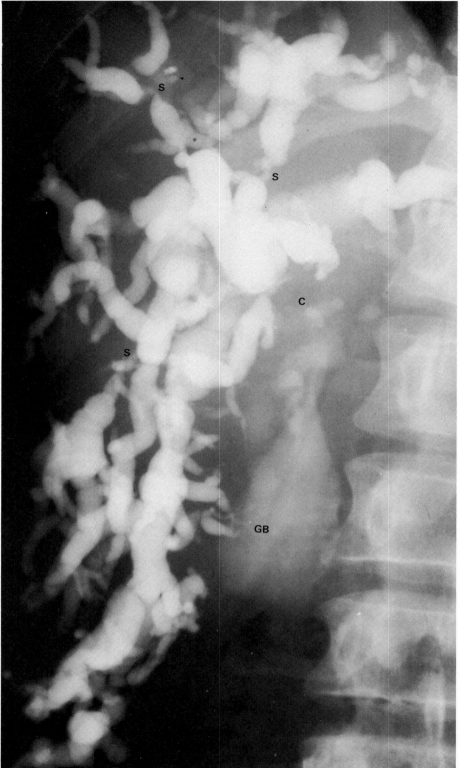

11.14 Cholangiocarcinoma in congenital hepatic fibrosis
Percutaneous cholangiogram The right, left and common hepatic ducts are obstructed *c*, although a small amount of contrast medium has passed the obstruction to outline the gallbladder *gb*. Though the intrahepatic ducts are dilated, there are short segments of narrowing *s*, which give the biliary tree an unusual configuration. At operation the obstruction was found to be due to cholangiocarcinoma, and a liver biopsy showed changes of congenital hepatic fibrosis (Courtesy of Dr. R.D. Dick)

11.14

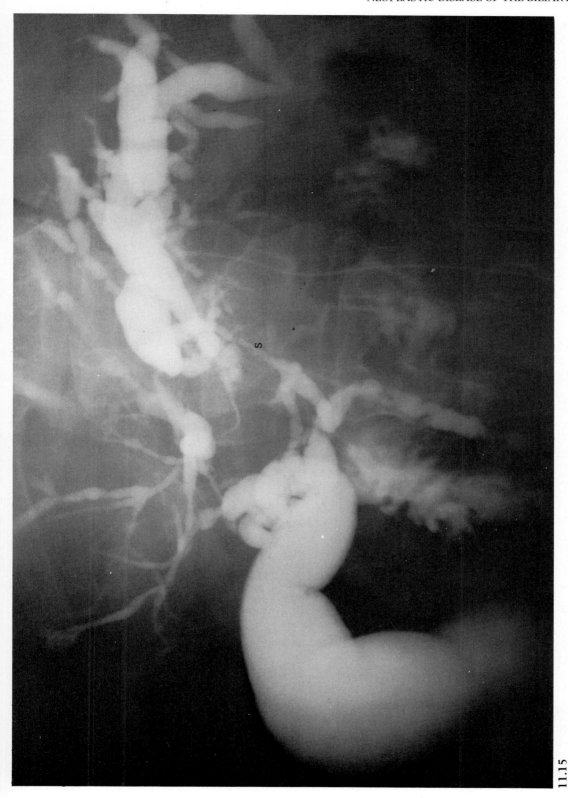

11.15

11.15 Sclerosing cholangitis and sclerosing carcinoma of the left hepatic duct A middle-aged man with long-standing ulcerative colitis developed bouts of jaundice and fever *Percutaneous cholangiogram* The catheter tip lies in a dilated duct in the left lobe of the liver proximal to a 3-cm-long stricture *s* of the left hepatic duct. The right intrahepatic ducts are displaced, irregular in outline but not dilated, and there is irregular narrowing of the common bile duct consistent with sclerosing cholangitis. At operation changes of sclerosing cholangitis in the common bile duct were confirmed but a sclerosing carcinoma causing stenosis of the left hepatic duct was found. Both conditions have an increased incidence in ulcerative colitis

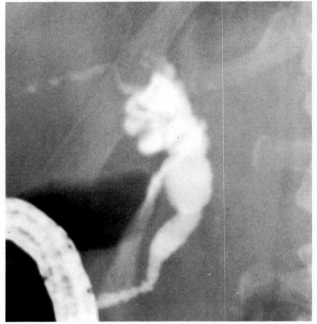

11.16a

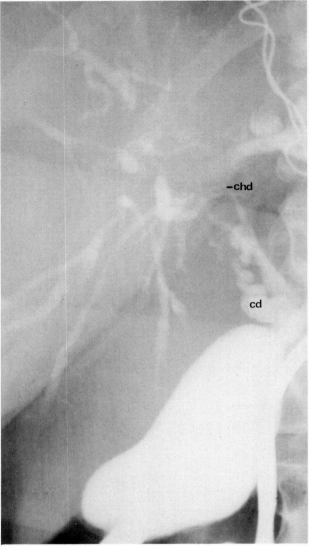

11.16b

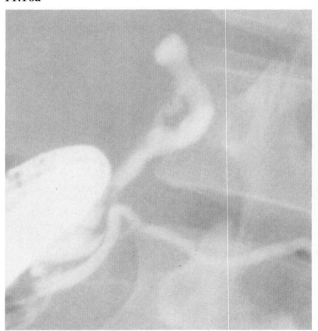

11.17

11.17 Enlarged lymph nodes at the porta hepatis An elderly woman who became jaundiced following colectomy for sigmoid carcinoma *Endoscopic cholangiogram and pancreatogram* There is abrupt occlusion of the common hepatic duct 1 cm above the insertion of the cystic duct. The pancreatic duct is normal in calibre and configuration

11.16 Sclerosing cholangitis and sclerosing cholangiocarcinoma A 45-year-old woman with long-standing ulcerative colitis developed progressive jaundice over a period of several months. a *Endoscopic cholangiogram* Irregular narrowing of the lower common bile duct and some proximal dilatation of the upper common bile and common hepatic duct is evident. Apart from an irregular narrowed duct in the right lobe, no intrahepatic duct filling could be achieved. b *Operative cholangiogram (3 months later)* Filling of the narrowed common hepatic duct *chd* and irregular but undilated ducts in the right lobe of the liver was achieved after forceful retrograde injection. Cystic duct *cd*. Biopsy of the common hepatic duct revealed cholangiocarcinoma and of the common bile duct revealed sclerosing cholangitis

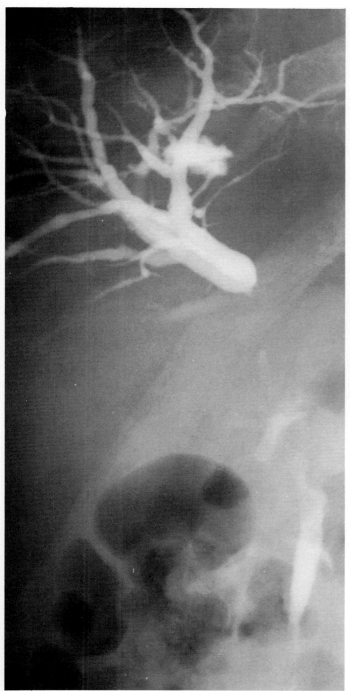

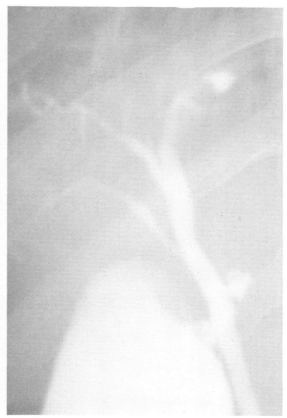

11.19

11.19 **Hepatoma** A 60-year-old Burmese man with liver failure and jaundice *Endoscopic cholangiogram* A small cavity filled with contrast medium from the left hepatic duct. The bile ducts are not dilated. At post-mortem there was cirrhosis of the liver with overlying hepatic carcinoma of multicentre origin. In places the liver had broken down into necrotic cystic areas

11.18

11.18 **Enlarged lymph nodes at the porta hepatis** A 68-year-old man with carcinomatosis from bronchial carcinoma *Percutaneous cholangiogram* The extrahepatic bile duct is narrowed for over 10 cm owing to compression by a mass of enlarged lymph nodes at the porta hepatis.

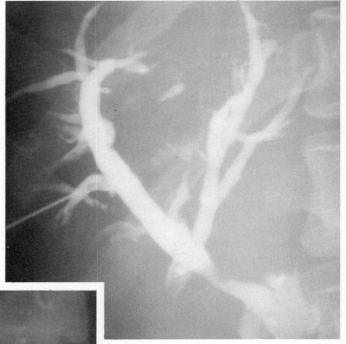

11.20

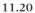

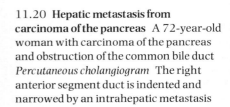

11.20 **Hepatic metastasis from
carcinoma of the pancreas** A 72-year-old
woman with carcinoma of the pancreas
and obstruction of the common bile duct
Percutaneous cholangiogram The right
anterior segment duct is indented and
narrowed by an intrahepatic metastasis

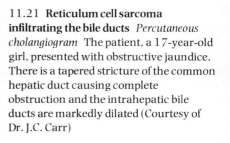

11.21 **Reticulum cell sarcoma
infiltrating the bile ducts** *Percutaneous
cholangiogram* The patient, a 17-year-old
girl, presented with obstructive jaundice.
There is a tapered stricture of the common
hepatic duct causing complete
obstruction and the intrahepatic bile
ducts are markedly dilated (Courtesy of
Dr. J.C. Carr)

11.21

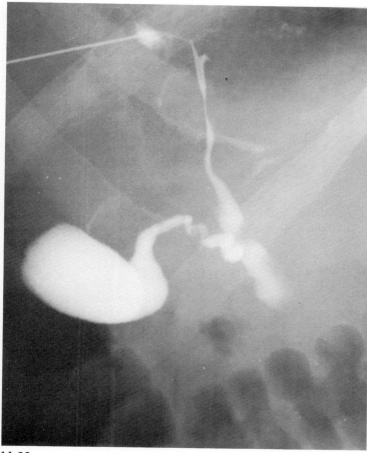

11.22

11.22 Cholangiocarcinoma The patient, a 62-year-old woman, had developed painless obstructive jaundice *Fine-needle cholangiography* There is narrowing of the common hepatic duct and obstruction at the junction of the right and left hepatic ducts

12 The Anatomy and Congenital Anomalies of the Pancreas

The pancreas lies retroperitoneally, roughly in the transpyloric plane, and for descriptive purposes is divided into the head, neck, body and tail. The head lies to the right or overlying the spine, within the duodenal loop, and the uncinate process projects from the lower part of the head posterior to the superior mesenteric vessels as these travel from behind the pancreas into the root of the mesentery. Posteriorly lie the inferior vena cava, aorta and crura of the diaphragm, the splenic artery runs along the upper border of the pancreas, and the splenic vein runs behind the gland to form the portal vein behind the pancreatic neck. The common bile duct lies either in a groove or embedded in the back of the head of the pancreas as it passes to the papilla of Vater. Anteriorly the stomach is separated by the lesser sac and the pancreatic tail lies against the hilum of the spleen.

The major arteries supplying branches to the pancreas are the gastro-duodenal, dorsal pancreatic, inferior pancreatico-duodenal arteries and the pancreatica magna and caudal pancreatic branches of the splenic artery. Although these arteries always arise from the coeliac or superior mesenteric arteries or their branches, there is a marked variation in their origin. The corresponding veins drain into the portal system.

The pancreas is lobulated and contained within a fine capsule. The lobules are made up of alveoli of secretory cells which drain via ductules into the principal ducts; between the alveoli lie the islets of Langerhans. The pancreas is usually oblique in position and sigmoid or L-shaped in configuration though in a minority of individuals it may be horseshoe-shaped or lie transversely (Kreel *et al.* 1973).

The pancreas is formed embryologically from ventral and dorsal pancreatic buds and the pattern of the main pancreatic ducts is determined by the arrangement of the ventral and dorsal pancreatic ducts. There are four major duct patterns (Dawson & Langman 1961).

1 In 40 per cent. of subjects the ventral duct and the dorsal duct in the body and tail of the gland unite to form the main pancreatic duct of Wirsung. The dorsal duct in the head of the pancreas, called Santorini's duct, remains patent, drains to the accessory papilla and may provide an alternative channel if the duct of Wirsung becomes obstructed near the papilla. Ampullary dilatation of the distal Santorini duct is often seen adjacent to the accessory papilla though it is uncommon at the papilla of Vater.

2 In 35 per cent. of subjects a combined duct is formed which drains the head, body and tail of the pancreas, but the accessory duct is obliterated either adjacent to the accessory papilla or adjacent to the main pancreatic duct so that there is no alternative channel.

3 Although in 17 per cent. of subjects the accessory duct is partly obliterated, an alternative channel, the ansa pancreatica, forms between the inferior branches of accessory and main pancreatic ducts in the lower part of the head. However, the calibre of the Santorini duct and the ansa pancreatica channel is sometimes very small and it has been considered that they could only function as alternative channels in 20 per cent. of subjects (Millbourn 1950). This accords with the authors' experience of retrograde pancreatography.

4 In 9 or 10 per cent of subjects the ventral and dorsal pancreatic ducts and their branches do not unite. The body and tail of the pancreas drain into the accessory papilla and the ventral duct drains to the biliary

papilla. The ventral duct has superior and inferior branches which drain the posterior portion of the head of the pancreas and the inferior branch of the dorsal duct drains the anterior aspect of the head of the pancreas. The size of the ventral portion of the pancreas may vary greatly.

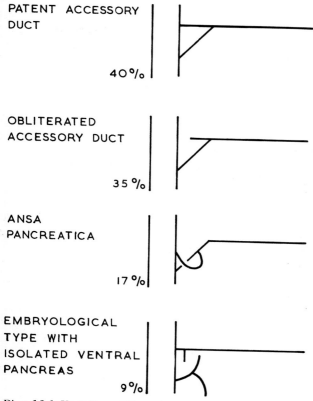

Diag. 12.1 Variations of the main pancreatic duct (after Dawson & Langman 1961)

Annular pancreas is a rare condition in which a band or ring of pancreatic tissue, continuous with the head of the gland, almost completely surrounds the second part of the duodenum; more than 100 cases have been reported (Dodd & Nafis 1956). It represents the ventral pancreatic bud which has not rotated normally and is drained by an isolated ventral duct system or its inferior branch. Other anomalies such as malrotation of the mid gut, oesophageal atresia or mongolism may be present (Gross 1953). Annular pancreas may be found at any level in the duodenum, although in the majority it occurs in the second part, and may present as duodenal obstruction in the new-born or be found incidentally at barium meal or post-mortem examination (Friedman 1957). In the infant a double bubble lucency may be evident on the erect abdomen film, and barium studies in the adult may show a localized smooth narrowing of the duodenum. Pancreatitis (Doubilet & Worth 1965) or carcinoma may develop within an annular pancreas.

Aberrant pancreatic tissue rests may occur anywhere in the duodenum or stomach; they present as intramural filling defects and at barium meal examination may be mistaken for benign tumours. Filling of a short duct may sometimes be evident (Eklof 1961) and ulceration may occur.

Unfortunately, the terms proximal and distal can have ambiguous connotations when describing retrograde studies, and the term caudad and cephalad may also be misunderstood. It is better to designate lesions as being in the head, body or tail of the pancreas, and to describe them as upstream or downstream of other features.

The calibre of the main duct has been measured in radiological studies of the normal pancreas at post-mortem examination (Millbourn 1950; Kreel *et al.* 1973). The post-mortem dimensions were on the whole greater than those observed in life and the age of the subjects was greater. Kreel *et al.* (1973) recorded that the width of the proximal part of the duct at post-mortem examination was less than 3 mm in only 26 per cent., 3–6 mm in 50 per cent. and 6–9 mm in 19 per cent. However, a duct calibre in excess of 6 mm in the head of the pancreas and 5 mm in the body should be viewed with suspicion when revealed in the retrograde or operative pancreatogram.

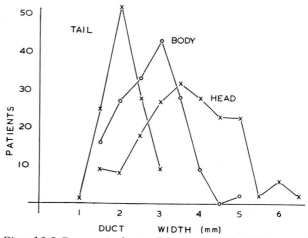

Diag. 12.2 Pancreatic duct widths measured in 178 normal endoscopic pancreatograms from Hannover, Erlangen, Brussels, London and Bristol (Cotton 1974)

The pancreatic duct may be indented by the superior mesenteric artery in the region of the body of the pancreas (Kreel *et al.* 1973), and the pattern of the side branches varies, usually with a long branch to the uncinate process and another to the upper portion of the head of the pancreas. The side branches in the body and tail of the gland are shorter than those in the head and may come off at right angles or obliquely to the main duct; they are normally slender, and third order branches are usually visible at retrograde pancreatography. Minimal ectasia of occasional side branches may be evident in the elderly, but is not a feature in normal adults. The main duct in the tail of the gland may be bifid. Like the common bile duct the pancreatic duct narrows as it passes through the duodenal wall.

The pancreatic and bile ducts have a common channel more than 3 mm long in over 50 per cent. of subjects and of less than 2 mm in about 30 per cent. of subjects (Dawson & Langman 1961). Separate orifices on the papilla are evident in 4 per cent. (Dowdy 1969). In the remaining 16 per cent. the pancreatic and bile ducts are separated by a thin septum to the papilla.

The normal pancreas secretes about one and one half litres of alkaline fluid per day, pancreatic enzymes being secreted by acinar cells and inorganic constituents secreted by cells lining the ducts. Secretin causes a profuse flow of pancreatic juice of high bicarbonate content whilst pancreozymin increases the enzyme content of pancreatic juice without increasing its volume. Aspiration of pancreatic juice from the duodenum, following injection of these hormones or the administration of a test meal, is used to assess the functional capacity of the pancreas.

References

Cotton P. (1974) *Endoscopy*, **6**, 65

Dawson W. & Langman J. (1961) *Anat. Rec.*, **139**, 59

Dodd G. D. & Nafis W. A. (1956) *Amer. J. Roentgenol.*, **75**, 333

Doubilet H. & Worth M. H. (1965) *Surgery*, **58**, 824

Dowdy G. S. Jnr. (1969) *The Biliary Tract*. Philadelphia: Lea & Febiger

Eklof O. (1961) *Acta chir. scand.*, **121**, 19

Friedman A. I. (1957) *Gastroenterology*, **32**, 1172

Gross R. E. (1953) *The Surgery of Infancy and Childhood*. Philadelphia: Saunders

Kreel L., Sandin B. & Slavin G. (1973) *Clin. Radiol.*, **24**, 154

Millbourn E. (1950) *Acta anat. (Basel)*, **9**, 1

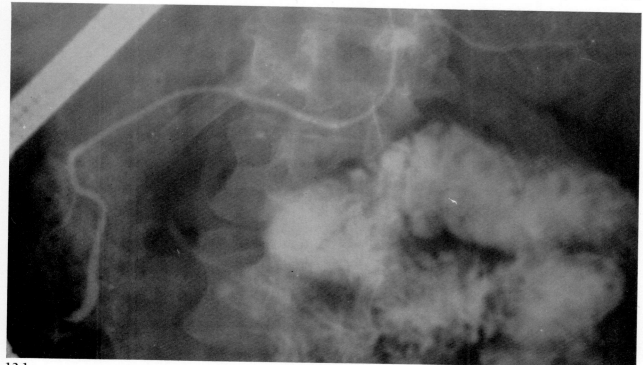

12.1

12.2

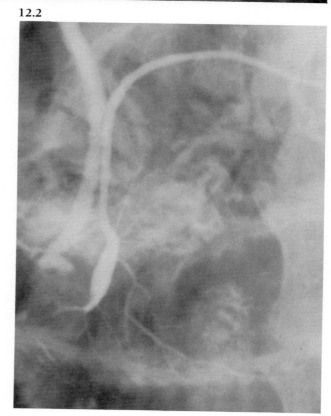

12.1 **Pancreatic duct** *Endoscopic pancreatogram* The main
duct is normal in calibre and sigmoid in configuration

12.2 **The duct to the uncinate process** *Endoscopic
pancreatogram* The duct system is shown after withdrawal
of the endoscope with the patient lying obliquely

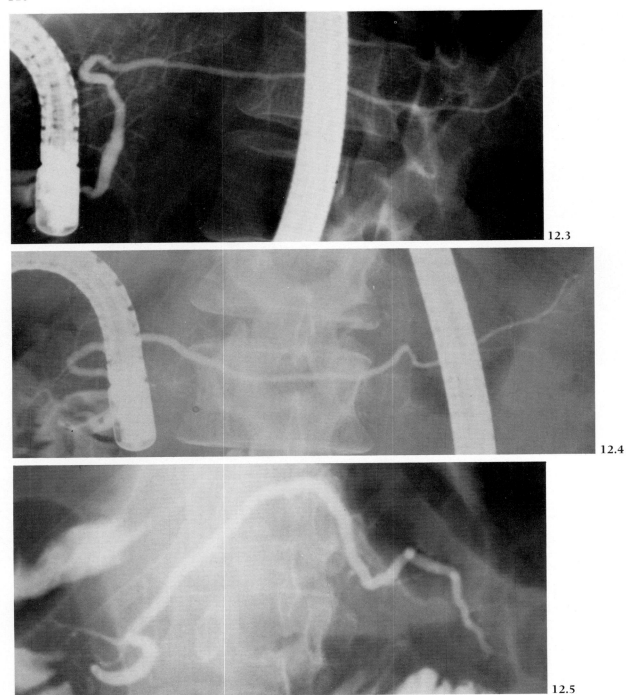

12.3 L-shaped pancreatic duct *Endoscopic pancreatogram* The slender side branches are well shown during retrograde injection

12.4 Transverse pancreas *Endoscopic pancreatogram*

12.5 Horseshoe configuration of the pancreas *Endoscopic pancreatogram*

12.6 **Vertical pancreas** *Endoscopic pancreatogram*
12.7 **Low pancreas** *Endoscopic cholangiogram* The body
and tail of the pancreas are below the head at the L4 level.
There is a large spleen displacing the tail of the pancreas
downward

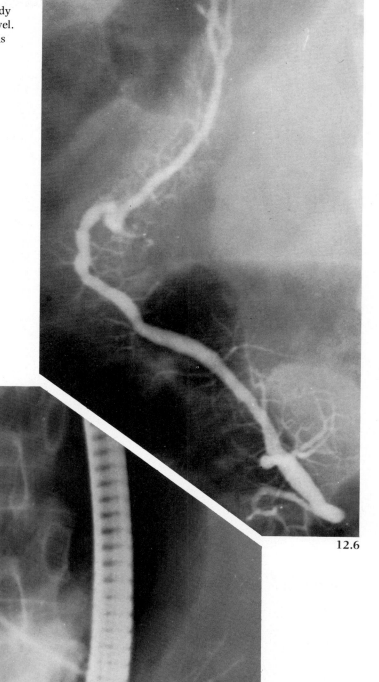

12.7

12.6

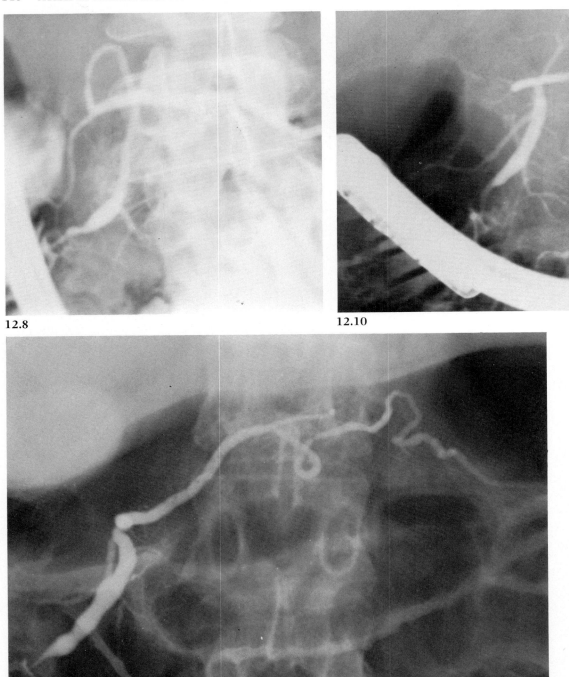

12.8

12.10

12.9

12.8 **Looped pancreatic duct** *Endoscopic pancreatogram* The main duct is looped in the region of the neck of the pancreas
12.9 **Looped pancreatic duct** *Endoscopic pancreatogram* The main duct is looped in the region of the body of the pancreas
12.10 **Blind Santorini duct** *Endoscopic pancreatogram* The blind end of the Santorini duct does not drain into the duodenum

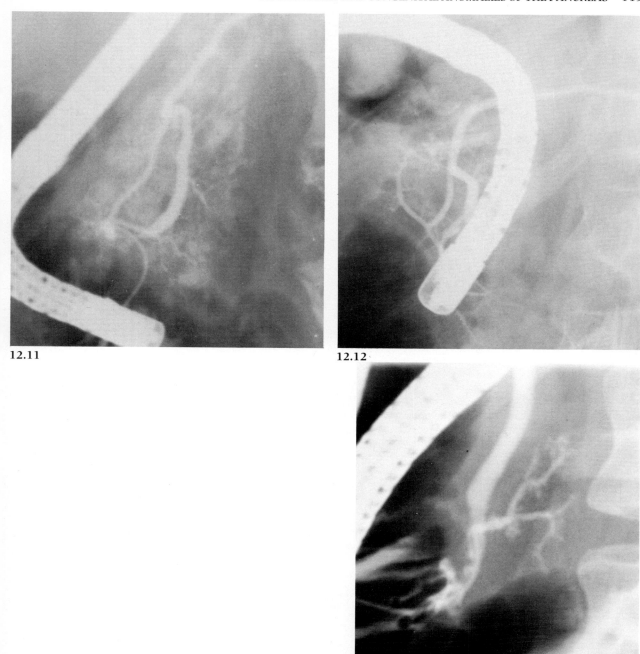

12.11

12.12

12.13

12.11 **Patent Santorini duct** *Endoscopic pancreatogram* The accessory papilla has been cannulated and the main pancreatic ducts have been filled with contrast agent. The duct from the lower part of the head is shown draining into the Santorini duct
12.12 **Ansa pancreatica** *Endoscopic pancreatogram*
12.13 **Isolated ventral pancreas** *Endoscopic pancreatogram and cholangiogram* The isolated ventral duct has superior and inferior branches, and drains to the papilla of Vater

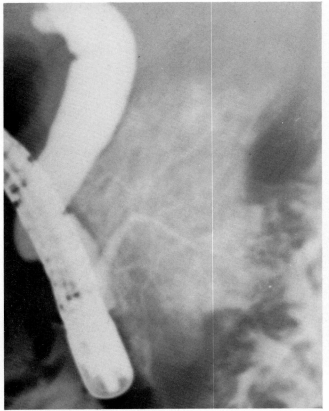

12.14

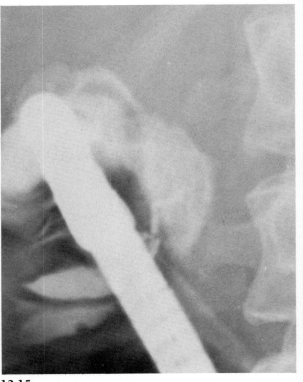

12.15

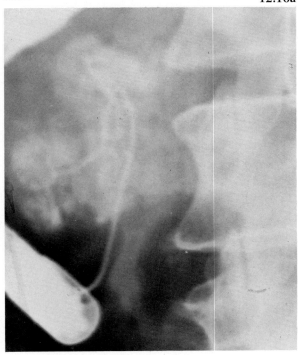

12.16a

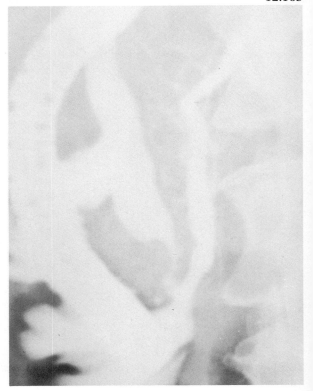

12.16b

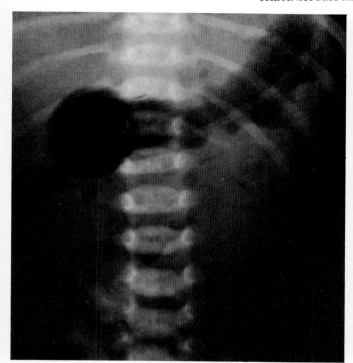

12.17a

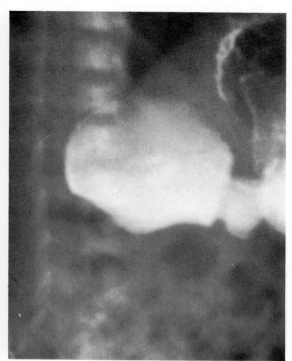

12.17b

12.17 Annular pancreas causing duodenal obstruction in a newborn infant a *Plain film* b *Barium meal* (Courtesy of Dr. I.R.S. Gordon)

Opposite page

12.14 Isolated ventral pancreas *Endoscopic pancreatogram and cholangiogram* A large ventral pancreas composes much of the head of the gland; acinar filling has occurred

12.15 Small isolated ventral pancreas *Endoscopic pancreatogram* Dense acinar filling partially obscures the small ventral duct system

12.16 Catheter tip in a side branch *Endoscopic pancreatogram* a The catheter has been advanced along the main duct with its tip in the duct to the upper part of the head of the pancreas. Acinar filling in the area supplied by the duct has occurred. b On withdrawal of the catheter into the common pancreatico-biliary channel; the main pancreatic and common bile ducts have filled well

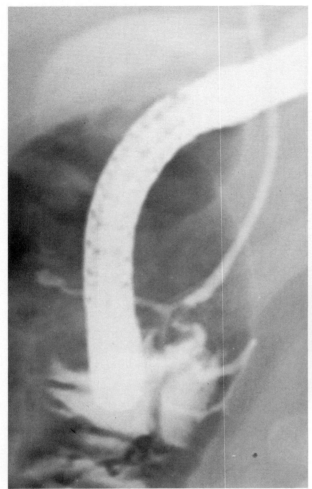

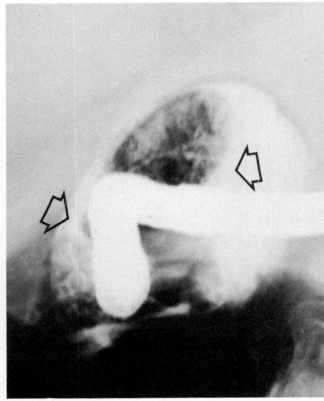

12.19

12.18

12.18 **Annular pancreas** *Endoscopic cholangiogram and pancreatogram* There is a long common channel, and pancreatic ducts extend medially and laterally around the descending duodenum. The lateral duct shows ampullary dilatation; the duodenum is not narrowed

12.19 **Annular pancreas** *Endoscopic pancreatogram* The catheter has been inserted into the papilla in the postero-medial aspect of the descending duodenum. The main duct draining the annular pancreas (arrows) curves posteriorly and laterally around the duodenum and is partially obscured by the endoscope, contrast medium in the duodenum and acini of the annular pancreas (Case referred by Mr. P. Huddy)

Acute pancreatitis

Acute pancreatitis is a clinical and biochemical syndrome in which recovery is usually associated with a return of structural and functional normality. Should the cause persist, relapsing acute pancreatitis, or in some cases progress to chronic pancreatitis with permanent change in the gland, may develop. Acute pancreatitis may be followed by sequelae such as abscess, pseudocyst or cicatricial stricture of the main pancreatic duct.

In Great Britain, acute pancreatitis is a relatively uncommon condition and the exact cause of many cases is unknown. About two-thirds of patients have biliary tract disease, a small proportion are alcoholics (Trapnell 1972), and there is an increased incidence in patients on steroids, women taking oral contraceptives and those with some forms of hyperlipaemia and hypercalcaemia. Pancreatic carcinoma and trauma may both produce pancreatitis.

Acute pancreatitis is an autodigestive disease in which digestive enzymes are released into the pancreatic tissues, and the pathological changes may range from mild cellular oedema to haemorrhagic necrosis. Peptidases seem to be the most damaging of the released enzymes, and lipase may produce fat necrosis. Serum amylase levels are elevated at an early stage in the disease in 90 per cent. of cases, but cholecystitis, bowel perforation and ischaemic lesions can also be associated with raised amylase levels. Serum lipase determinations may be helpful in these cases, and a fall in the serum calcium level indicates significant fat necrosis, often associated with a poor prognosis.

Patients usually present as acute abdominal emergencies, but relapsing cases tend to be less severe. Although in half the patients the course is relatively mild, there is an overall mortality rate of 10–20 per cent. which increases with age (Trapnell 1972). Ventilation–perfusion changes in the lungs causing anoxia contribute significantly to the death rate.

Haematemesis due to associated duodenal ulceration or from haemoductal pancreatitis may occur. Pseudocysts which have no epithelial lining result from extravasation of pancreatic enzymes into the interstitial tissues; they project between the liver and stomach or into the lesser sac as encapsulated effusions, and may contain clear fluid, altered blood or necrotic tissue. Abscess formation may occur. Duodenal ileus and wound dehiscence are common following laparotomy. Pulmonary collapse and pleural effusion are more common on the left side. Bone infarction due to fat necrosis may occur (Immelman *et al.* 1964).

Chronic pancreatitis Most patients with chronic pancreatitis present with abdominal pain which may radiate to the back and which is relieved in anteflexion. Lying on the back may increase the pain which tends to be recurrent with intervals of days or months between attacks. Loss of weight occurs commonly in association with pain. A small proportion of patients may have no pain and may present with diabetes, steatorrhoea or apyrexial jaundice.

Chronic pancreatitis or relapsing chronic pancreatitis, if the clinical course is marked by acute exacerbations, is characterized by residual

13 Pancreatitis

pancreatic damage which persists even if the causative factors are removed (Sarles *et al.* 1965).

Whilst biliary disease, peptic ulceration and mesenteric ischaemia may produce a similar clinical picture, the most difficult diagnosis is between chronic pancreatitis and pancreatic carcinoma.

Patients with chronic pancreatitis are mainly males who tend to be younger than those with acute pancreatitis and who have a mean age at onset of 38 years (Sarles *et al.* 1965). Calcifying pancreatitis occurs more commonly where the incidence of alcoholism is high and excessive alcoholic intake is the major aetiological factor. Protein malnutrition is a major cause of calcifying pancreatitis in tropical countries (Shaper 1960), although there is no evidence that protein malnutrition is associated with alcoholic pancreatitis in Europe. Hereditary pancreatitis occurring as an autosomal disorder and presenting in childhood has been described (Whitten *et al.* 1968). Pancreatitis occurs in 3–6 per cent. of patients with hyperparathyroidism (Herskovic *et al.* 1967), and alpha-1-antitrypsin deficiency has been observed in a high proportion of patients with chronic pancreatitis (Brunt 1975). Recurrent bouts of pancreatitis occurring in association with gallstones are probably examples of progression of acute pancreatitis due to persistent cholelithiasis.

Severe impairment of pancreatic function occurs in about 80 per cent. of children with mucoviscidosis (di Sant'Agnese & Talamo 1967) and calcifying chronic pancreatitis has been described in the relatives of patients with this disorder.

The main pathological finding in human and experimental chronic pancreatitis is the presence of protein plugs in the ducts, some of which are calcified. The parenchyma is replaced by dilated ducts and fibrosis. Strictures, dilatation and concrements in the main pancreatic duct occur late in the disease process. Retention cyst formation due to obstruction of the pancreatic ducts, acute pancreatitis with haemorrhagic necrosis and pseudocyst formation may also be present.

Radiology

Acute pancreatitis   On the plain abdomen film dilated gas-filled small bowel loops may be seen as 'sentinel loops' in the region of the pancreas. Air in the duodenal loop may reveal an 'epsilon' configuration of the medial aspect of the descending duodenum because of oedematous enlargement of the head of pancreas. Gas and faeces may be retained in the right side of the colon because of localized ileus in the transverse colon, and gas formation within the necrotic pancreas or a pancreatic abscess may produce pancreatic emphysema (Baylin & Weeks 1944). Oedema in the pancreas may be observed as a wedge-shaped opacity between the gastric antrum and the transverse colon. Further radiological studies are not usually necessary although barium meal examination may reveal oedematous thickening of the duodenal mucosa and enlargement of the duodenal loop. Thickened oedematous folds may be evident on the posterior aspect of the body of the stomach (Frimann-Dahl 1960) and plaques of calcification may develop in areas of fat necrosis which occur following acute pancreatitis.

Pseudocyst or abscess formation may present as a mass and can be localized by barium meal studies as a filling defect or displacement of the stomach, duodenal loop or transverse colon. Calcification may be evident in the wall of pancreatic pseudocysts (Waugh & Lynn 1958). Intravenous urography may reveal displacement of the kidneys and ureters (Atkinson *et al.* 1973). Endoscopic pancreatography is contraindicated until three weeks after an episode of acute pancreatitis because it may cause exacerbation. Prompt homogeneous opacification of the pancreatic parenchyma after injection of only a few millilitres of contrast medium has been seen in a few patients who have been examined during an attack. Cholelithiasis may later be demonstrated by cholangiography in over 50 per cent. of cases, and common duct calculi are present in about 10 per cent. (Guien 1972).

Chronic pancreatitis   Calcified concrements may be present in the pancreatic ducts in advanced chronic pancreatitis and these are evident on the plain abdomen films in about 10–20 per cent. of cases in the United Kingdom; the incidence of calcification is much higher in some other countries (Guien 1972). Tomography and oblique abdomen views may be necessary to reveal more subtle calcifications partly obscured by the spine.

The barium meal signs of chronic pancreatitis are shown best at hypotonic duodenography. The earliest sign is of flattening of the medial margin of the duodenal loop; the medial aspects of the circular folds are obliterated and the medial wall of the duodenum may show an epsilon configuration similar to that seen with pancreatic carcinoma. The first part of the duodenum may also be compressed and deformed by chronic pancreatitis, but the distinction between it and deformity due to past duodenal ulceration may be difficult. Coexistent duodenal ulceration is commonly present.

Endoscopic pancreatography shows changes in the main pancreatic duct and its major side branches as a result of chronic pancreatitis. These have been graded into 'minimal', 'moderate' and 'advanced' changes (Kasugai *et al.* 1972).

Minimal change pancreatitis is characterized by dilatation and shortening of side ducts with poor filling of the third and fourth order ducts; the side ducts may be irregular in direction but the main pancreatic duct is normal in calibre and configuration. In moderate change pancreatitis there is stricturing and irregular dilatation of the main pancreatic duct in addition to side duct changes. Advanced change pancreatitis indicates main duct obstruction, retention cyst formation and duct concrements.

There is good correlation between the pancreatogram signs of chronic pancreatitis and the pancreatic function tests, and the pancreatic scintiscan will show impaired uptake in over 95 per cent. of subjects with pancreatographic evidence of pancreatitis (Salmon *et al.* 1975).

Cholangiography reveals biliary calculi far less often in patients with chronic pancreatitis than in those with acute pancreatitis. Tapering strictures of the retropancreatic bile ducts are evident in about half the patients with advanced chronic pancreatitis, and there is usually moderate dilatation of the bile ducts above the obstruction. Pseudocysts and retention cysts may compress or displace the bile ducts and gallbladder.

Angiography is rarely used as a primary diagnostic procedure, but the changes seen in pancreatitis are important in the differentiation from carcinoma. The major intrapancreatic arteries show beaded dilatation and hypervascularity manifested by an increase in the number of arterial branches and an increased accumulation of contrast medium during the capillary phase. Small aneurysms may be demonstrated (White *et al.* 1976). The normal course of the arteries is unchanged, unlike the abrupt angulations and distortions of carcinoma. The encasements of vessels in carcinoma tend to be irregular and jagged whereas narrowing in chronic pancreatitis is smooth and even. The overall vascularity is decreased in carcinoma.

If a pseudocyst is present there may be stretching of arteries around the lesion. Very small retention cysts displace only the intrapancreatic branches, but large cysts may displace the splenic, hepatic, gastroduodenal and mesenteric arteries. Even a large cyst may cause only minimal vascular displacement if it lies anterior to the pancreas (Reuter *et al.* 1969).

References

Atkinson G. O., Clements J. L. Jnr., Milledge R. D. & Weens H. S. (1973) *Clin. Radiol.*, **24**, 185

Baylin G. J. & Weeks K. D. (1944) *Radiology*, **42**, 466

Brunt P. W. (1976) In *Modern Trends in Gastroenterology*, (Ed. Read A.E.) p. 134. London: Butterworths

di Sant'Agnese P. A. & Talamo R. C. (1967) *New Engl. J. Med.*, **277**, 1287

Frimann-Dahl J. (1960) *Roentgen Examinations in Acute Abdominal Diseases*. Springfield Illinois: Thomas

Guien C. (1972) *Clin. Gastroent.*, **1**, 61

Herskovic T., Keating F. R. Jnr. & Gross J. B. (1967) *Gastroenterology*, **52**, 1093

Immelman E. J., Bank S., Krige H. & Marks I. N. (1964) *Amer. J. Med.*, **36**, 96

Kasugai T., Kuno N., Kizu M., Koboyashi S. & Hattori K. (1972) *Gastroenterology*, **63**, 227

Reuter S. R., Redman H. C. & Joseph R. R. (1969) *Amer. J. Roentgenol.*, **107**, 56

Sarles H., Sarles J.-C., Camatte R., Muratore R., Gaini M., Guien C., Pastor J. & Le Roy F. (1965) *Gut*, **6**, 545

Shaper A. G. (1960) *Lancet*, **i**, 1223

Salmon P. R., Baddeley H., Machado G., Low-Beer T., Rhys-Davies E. & Trapnell J. (1975) *Gut*, **16**, 830

Trapnell J. (1972) *Clin. Gastroent.*, **1**, 147

Waugh J. M. & Lynn T. E. (1958) *Arch. Surg.*, **77**, 47

White A. F., Baum S. & Buranasiri S. (1976) *Amer. J. Roentgenol.*, **127**, 393

Whitten D. M., Feingold M. & Eisenklam E. J. (1968) *Amer. J. Dis. Child.*, **116**, 426

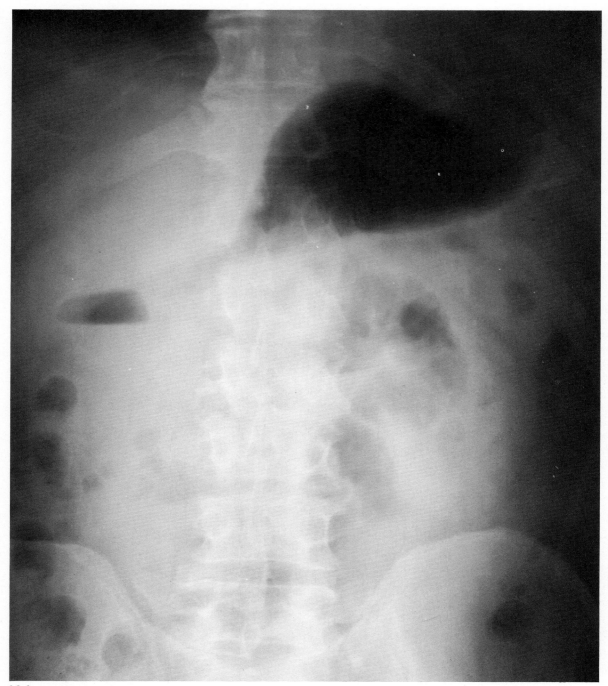

13.1

13.1 **Acute pancreatitis** *Plain abdomen* Several gas-distended, 'sentinel' small bowel loops are shown in the centre of the abdomen and there is upward displacement of the body and antrum of the stomach
Opposite page 13.2 **Resolving acute pancreatitis** *Endoscopic pancreatogram* Prompt homogeneous opacification of the pancreatic parenchyma has occurred following the injection of 2 or 3 ml of Angiografin. The side branches are poorly defined. Parenchymal filling in a normal pancreas occurs after the injection of much larger quantities of contrast medium and has an irregular lobular distribution

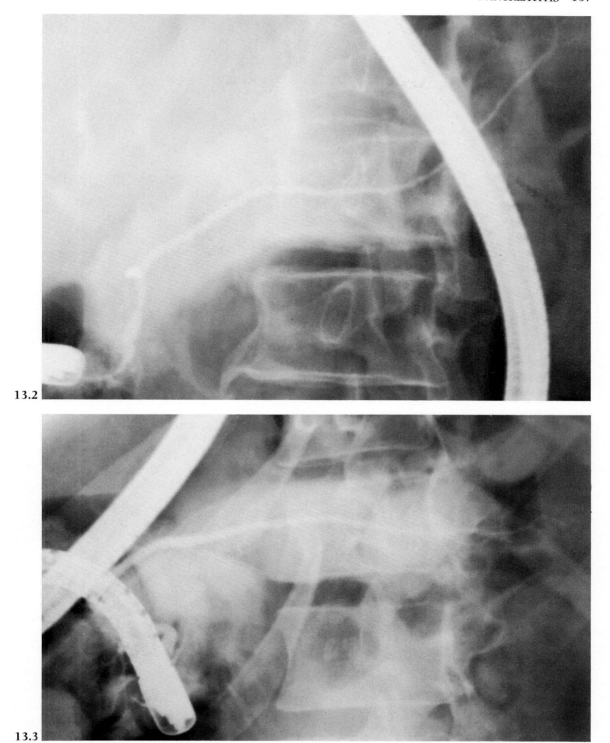

13.3 **Acute pancreatitis** *Endoscopic pancreatogram* Prompt homogeneous parenchymal filling in the body and tail of the pancreas

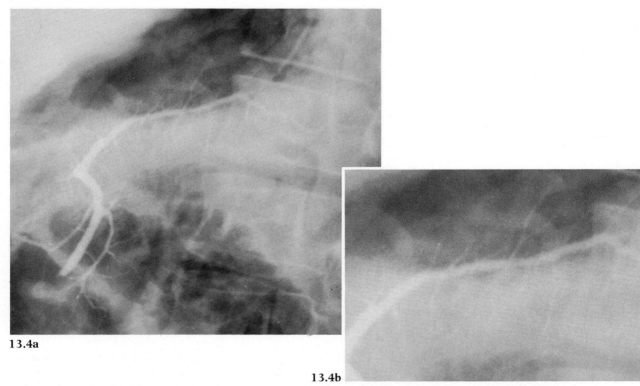

13.4a

13.4b

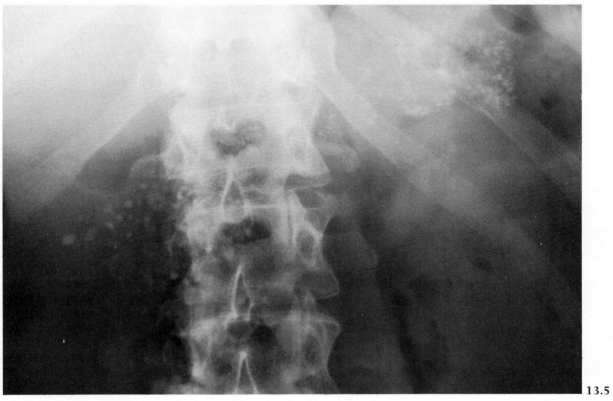

13.5

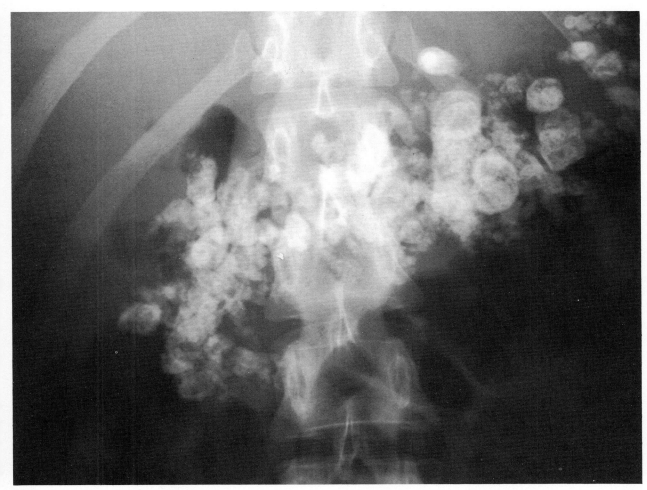

13.6

13.6 **Chronic pancreatitis** *Plain abdomen* Numerous calcified concrements are present throughout the pancreas, some of which are over 2 cm in diameter

Opposite page
13.4 **Acute relapsing pancreatitis**   This 40-year-old seaman had suffered well-documented bouts of acute pancreatitis in nearly every port from Southampton to Hong Kong, yet pancreatography and pancreatic function tests were normal eight weeks after his last attack *Endoscopic pancreatogram* a The main pancreatic duct is normal in calibre and configuration, and the side branches in the body of the pancreas b (close-up) taper and branch normally
13.5 **Chronic pancreatitis** *Plain abdomen* Multiple small opacities are shown in the upper abdomen due to calcified concrements throughout the pancreas

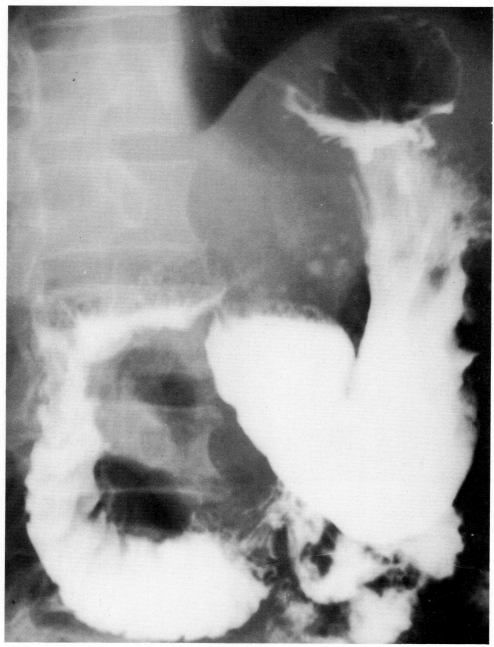

13.7

13.7 Chronic pancreatitis in a Ugandan—probably nutritional *Barium meal* The wall of the descending duodenum is indented along its medial aspect and there are calcified pancreatic concrements behind the stomach

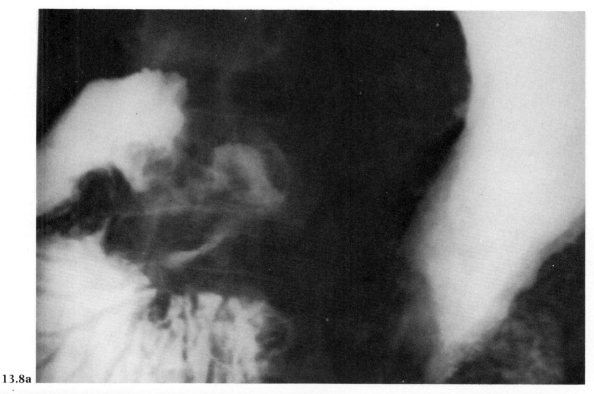

13.8a

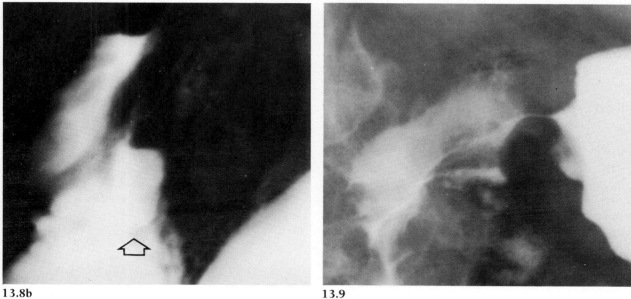

13.8b   **13.9**

13.8 Giant duodenal ulcer penetrating the pancreas and chronic pancreatitis *Barium meal* a The duodenal cap has been replaced by a giant ulcer crater, pancreatic calcification is evident.   b Lateral view of the first part of the duodenum showing the large ulcer projecting posteriorly into the pancreas (arrow)

13.9 Chronic pancreatitis *Barium meal (coned view of the first part of duodenum)* The pylorus is narrowed and elongated and there are filling defects in the duodenal cap due to extrinsic impression by the enlarged pancreas. Concrements are present in the head of the pancreas

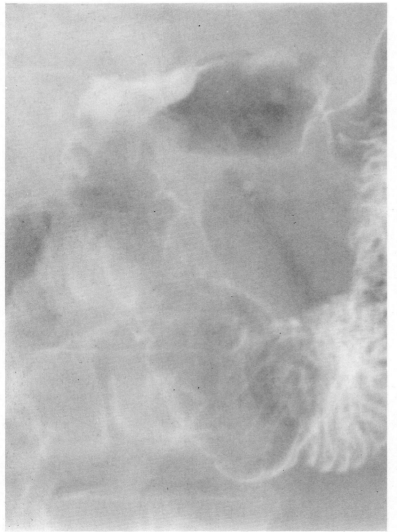

13.10

13.10 **Chronic pancreatitis** *Tubeless hypotonic duodenography (Buscopan I.V.)* The medial wall of the descending duodenum is indented above and below the papilla by the enlarged pancreas to give the 'reversed 3' or 'epsilon' sign. This configuration is thought to be due to traction on the papilla by the common bile duct and main pancreatic ducts and may be seen in inflammatory and neoplastic disease of the pancreas

Opposite page
13.11 **Chronic pancreatitis** *Endoscopic pancreatogram* The main pancreatic duct is irregular in calibre throughout its length. There is some narrowing in the tail, and the side branches are short, stubby and narrowed adjacent to their insertion into the main duct
13.12 **Chronic pancreatitis** *Endoscopic pancreatogram* There is beaded dilatation of the main pancreatic duct proximal to a 2-cm long stricture above the papilla. The side ducts throughout the pancreas are dilated and distorted even in the region of the stricture. The latter feature is indicative of inflammatory rather than neoplastic stricture

13.11

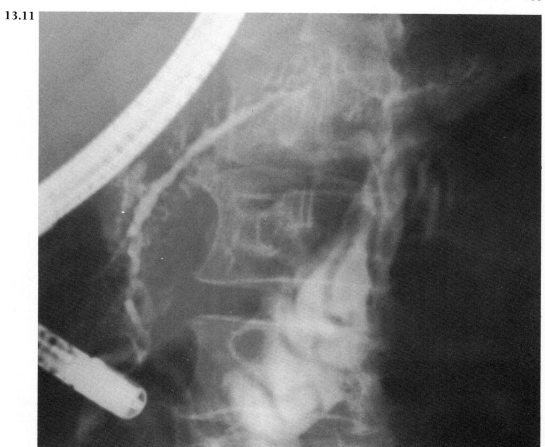

13.12

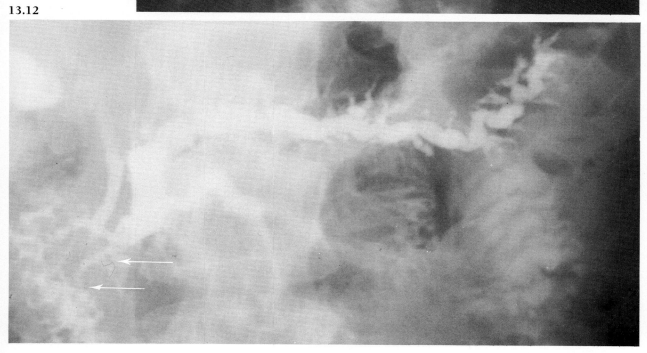

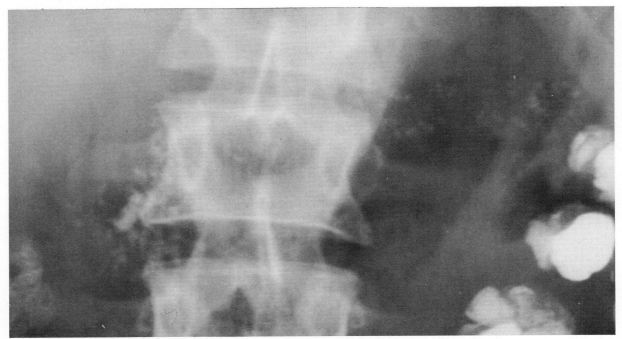

13.13a

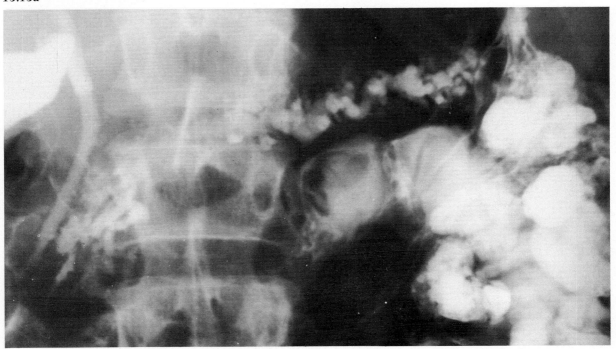

13.13b

13.13 **Chronic pancreatitis** a *Plain film* Nodular calcification is present throughout the pancreas and there is residual barium in the colon following barium meal examination. b *Endoscopic pancreatogram* The pancreatic ducts are dilated and irregular. The pancreatic calcification is obscured, indicating that it is due to calcified concrements in the ducts and not to parenchymal calcification

13.14 Chronic pancreatitis *Endoscopic pancreatogram* The main pancreatic duct is grossly dilated and looks like a string of short sausages. There are several lucent concrements in the pancreatic duct

13.15   **13.14**

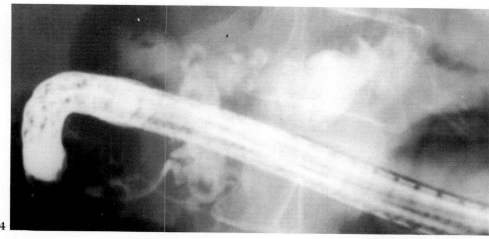

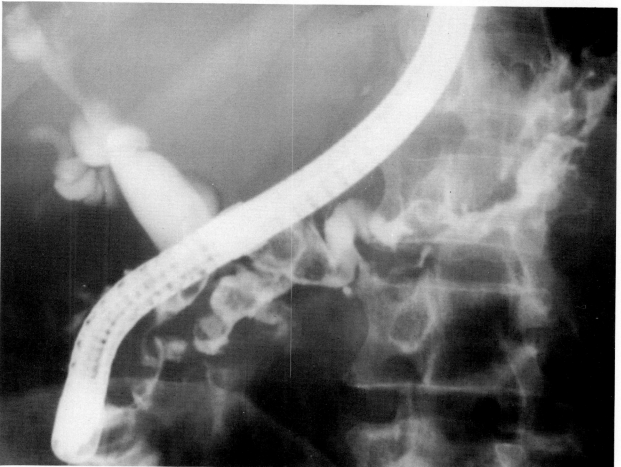

13.15 Chronic pancreatitis with common bile duct stricture *Endoscopic cholangiogram and pancreatogram* The main pancreatic duct is dilated and contains a number of lucent concrements. There is a stricture of the lower common bile duct with irregular dilatation of the biliary tree above, and short strictures of the right hepatic, common hepatic and upper common bile ducts due to ascending cholangitis

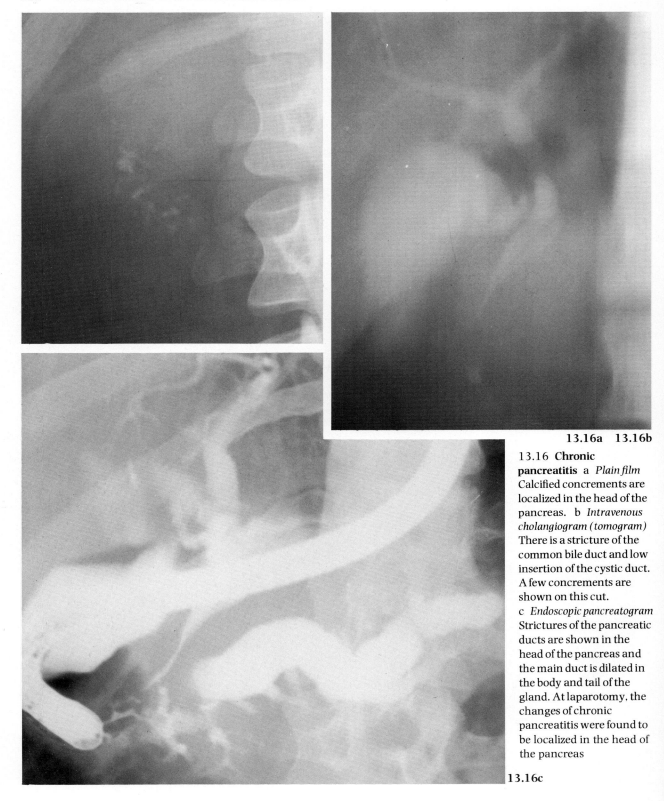

13.16a   13.16b

13.16 **Chronic pancreatitis** a *Plain film* Calcified concrements are localized in the head of the pancreas. b *Intravenous cholangiogram (tomogram)* There is a stricture of the common bile duct and low insertion of the cystic duct. A few concrements are shown on this cut. c *Endoscopic pancreatogram* Strictures of the pancreatic ducts are shown in the head of the pancreas and the main duct is dilated in the body and tail of the gland. At laparotomy, the changes of chronic pancreatitis were found to be localized in the head of the pancreas

13.16c

13.17 **Stricture of the main pancreatic duct due to chronic pancreatitis** *Endoscopic pancreatogram* There is an area of narrowing in the body of the pancreas; a small dilated side duct is present adjacent to the stricture, and side duct ectasia is evident downstream in the head of the pancreas. These features favour an inflammatory rather than a neoplastic stricture

13.18 **Drainage of obstructed pancreatic duct to the stomach** *Endoscopic pancreatogram* Dilated pancreatic duct, ectatic side ducts and a stricture in the body of the gland due to chronic pancreatitis are shown. Contrast medium has entered the stomach through a caudal pancreatico-gastrostomy

13.19 **Obstructed pancreatic duct due to a large concrement** The patient presented with steatorrhoea and abdominal pain of abrupt onset *Endoscopic cholangiogram and pancreatogram* Pancreatic calcification was present on the plain film, but pancreatography confirmed that there was obstruction of the main pancreatic duct in the head by an impacted concrement

13.19

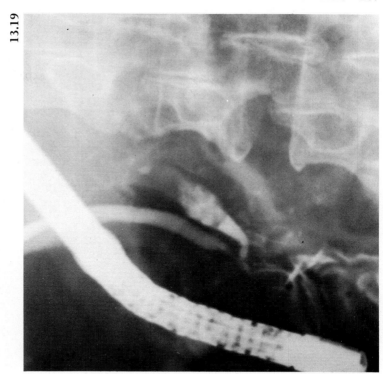

13.18

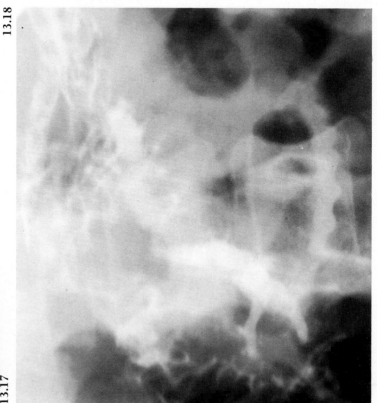

13.17

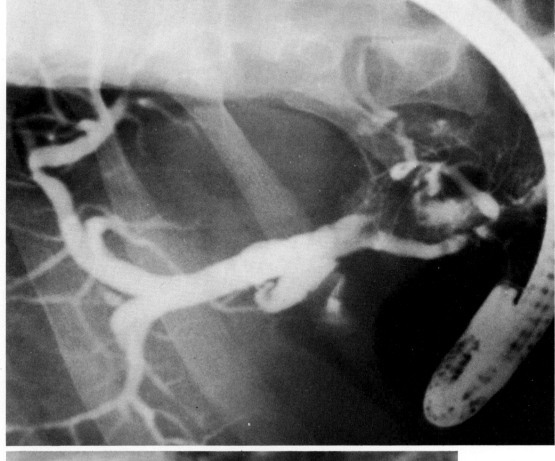

13.20

13.20   Multiple strictures of the main pancreatic duct due to pancreatitis *Endoscopic cholangiogram and pancreatogram* A stricture of the main duct is apparent 3 cm above the papilla. The duct above this obstruction is undilated, irregular in calibre and shows poor side duct filling, and it is totally obstructed in the body of the pancreas. The occurrence of two or more strictures with patent duct between them indicates the presence of pancreatitis, although coexistent carcinoma cannot be excluded

13.21

13.21   Obstruction of the main pancreatic duct due to pancreatitis *Endoscopic cholangiogram and pancreatogram* The main pancreatic duct shows tapered obstruction in the body of the pancreas. However, there are several ectatic side ducts in the head of the pancreas where the main duct is narrowed, and the lower common bile duct is narrowed. The presence of side duct ectasia and the distribution of the changes favoured a diagnosis of chronic pancreatitis which was confirmed at laparotomy

13.22 Chronic pancreatitis *Endoscopic pancreatogram* Dilatation of the main pancreatic duct is shown in the head of the pancreas (10 mm) but despite good filling of the main duct there is very sparse filling of side ducts in the body of the pancreas

13.23 Chronic pancreatitis *Endoscopic cholangiogram and pancreatogram* The main duct in the body of the pancreas is dilated (6 mm). There is good filling of side branches, which are irregular in direction, shortened and stubby in the body and tail of the pancreas. The term 'minimal change pancreatitis' has been applied to this appearance

13.24 Chronic pancreatitis with changes localized to the side ducts *Endoscopic cholangiography and pancreatography* The main pancreatic duct is normal in calibre, but the side ducts in the body of the gland are stubby and show poor filling of the third order ducts. There is narrowing of the lower common bile duct due to pancreatitis in the head

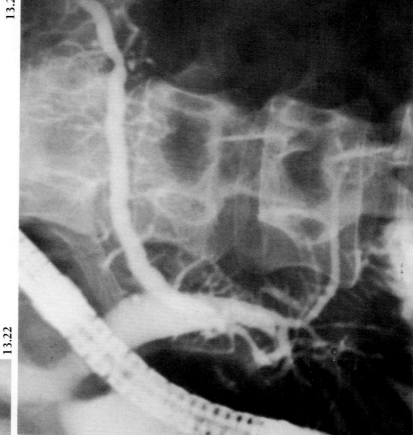

13.23

13.22

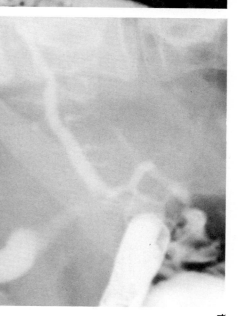

13.24

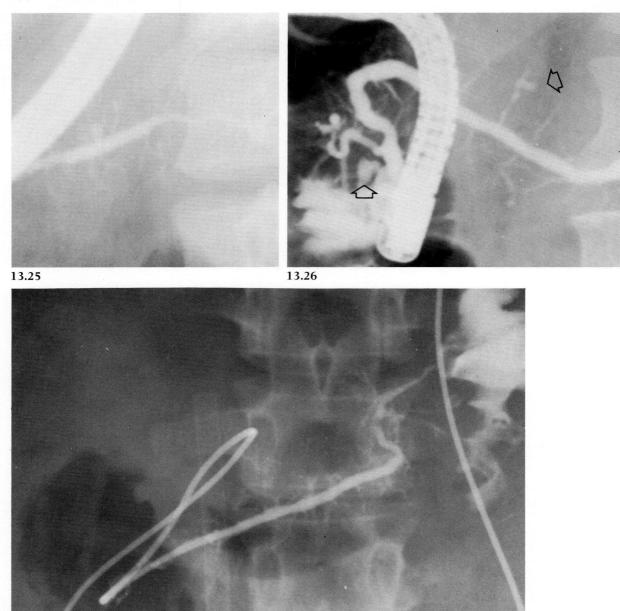

13.25

13.26

13.27

13.25 Chronic pancreatitis producing side duct ectasia in the absence of change in the main pancreatic ducts *Pancreatogram with detailed views of the body of the pancreas* Some side ducts are normal in configuration, but several above the main duct show ectasia and poor filling of third order ducts

13.26 Chronic pancreatitis *Endoscopic pancreatogram* Side-duct ectasia (arrowed) is seen

13.27 Chronic pancreatitis *Operative pancreatogram prior to pancreatectomy* The catheter has been inserted into the main pancreatic duct following caudal pancreatectomy. The main duct is normal in calibre and configuration but the side ducts are stunted consistent with the operative findings of a shrunken pancreas

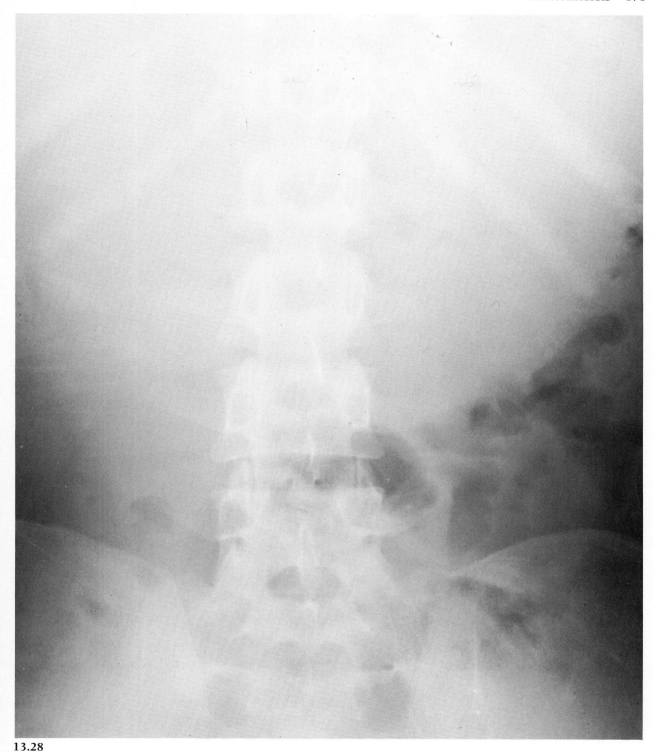

13.28

13.28 Pancreatic pseudocyst *Plain abdomen (supine)* There is a large soft tissue mass in the epigastrium due to a large pseudocyst whose lower border is outlined by gas in the transverse colon

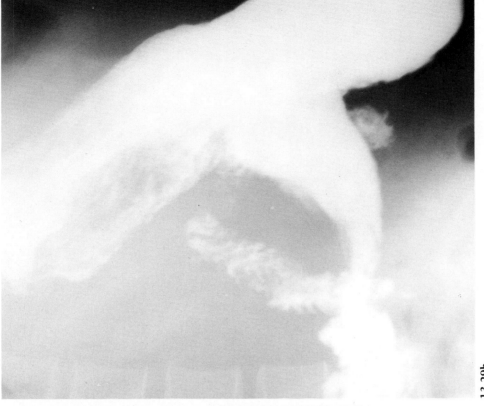

13.29b

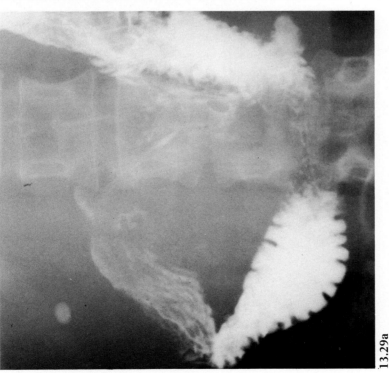

13.29a

13.29 Recurrent pancreatitis and pseudocyst a *Barium meal (AP)* The gastric antrum and duodenal bulb are deformed and flattened by the pseudocyst. The calcified stone indicates the position of the gallbladder. b *Barium meal (lateral)* The body of the stomach is displaced forwards and the gastric antrum is stretched around the cyst. c *Oral cholecystogram* The gallbladder which contains an opaque calculus is indented medially by a large pseudocyst. Pancreatic concrements are evident

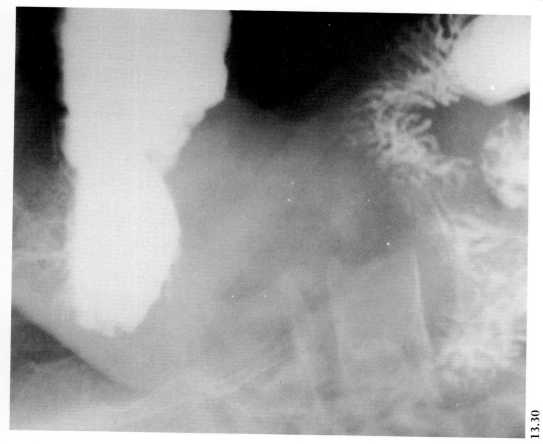

13.30

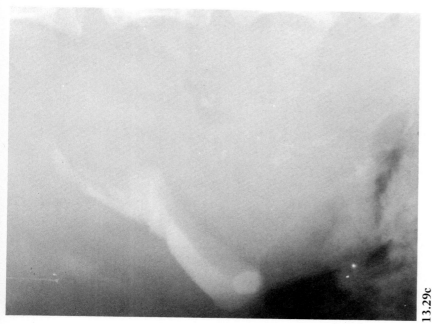

13.29c

13.30 Pseudocyst *Barium meal (lateral)* A large cyst is displacing the stomach upwards and forwards. The duodenal loop is widened and compressed

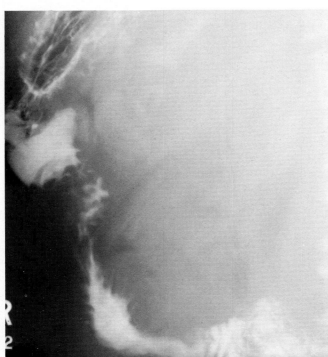

13.31a

13.31 **Pancreatic pseudocyst before and after surgical drainage** a *Barium meal and intravenous cholangiogram (before operation)* The duodenal loop is compressed and displaced forward by the pseudocyst. The dilated common hepatic duct is opacified. b *Barium meal following choledochoduodenostomy and cystojejunostomy* Barium has filled a large triangular pseudocyst cavity via the cystojejunostomy and has entered the intrahepatic ducts via the choledochoduodenostomy. c *Barium meal (lateral)* The dependent portion of the cavity is outlined by barium and is shown to lie behind the stomach and duodenum

13.31b

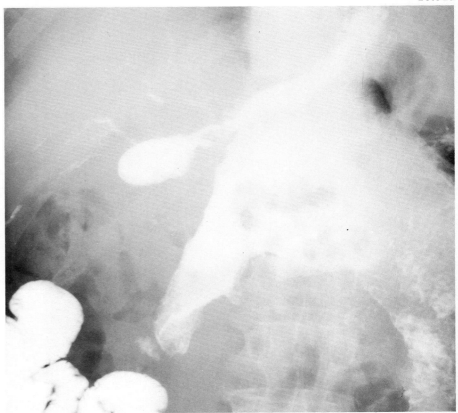

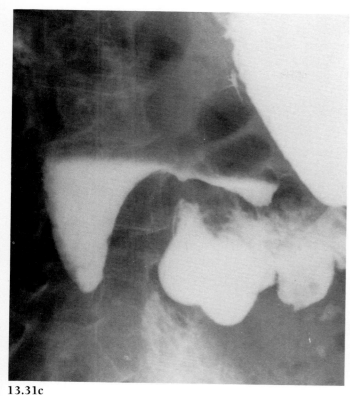

13.31c

13.32 **Chronic pancreatitis with retention cysts** *Endoscopic pancreatogram* The main pancreatic duct is irregular in calibre, and side-duct ectasia is present. Three large, smooth-walled cysts are filled with contrast medium

13.32

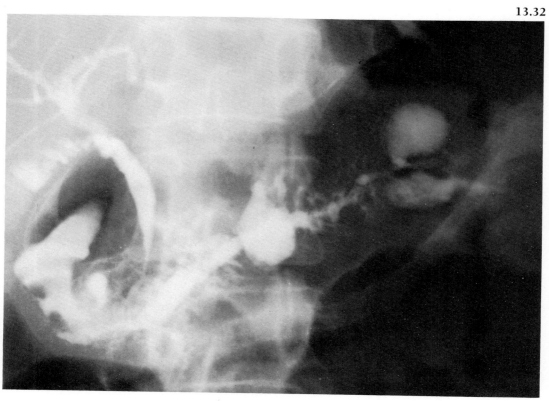

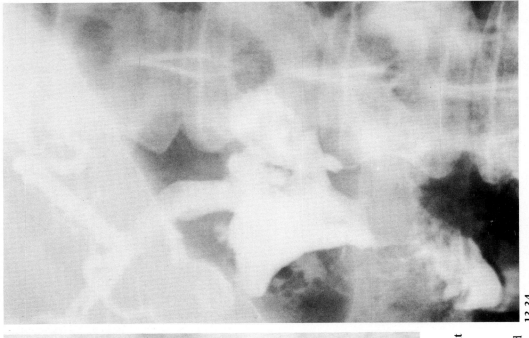

13.33

13.34

13.33 Small cavity in the head of the pancreas following an acute exacerbation of recurrent pancreatitis *Endoscopic pancreatogram* The pancreatic ducts show minor changes, and a small irregular cavity has filled with contrast medium (arrow)

13.34 Palpable pseudocyst following acute pancreatitis *Endoscopic pancreatogram and cholangiogram* The papilla was cannulated normally and a large irregular cavity in the head of the pancreas has been outlined. The biliary tree appears normal but there is no filling of the main pancreatic duct in the body and tail

13.35 Pseudocyst in the head of the pancreas compressing the lower common bile duct *Endoscopic cholangiogram and pancreatogram* The lowest 5 cm of the common bile duct are indented and displaced. There is obstruction of the pancreatic duct in the body of the pancreas and a lobulated cavity in the region of the bile duct has been faintly outlined with contrast medium

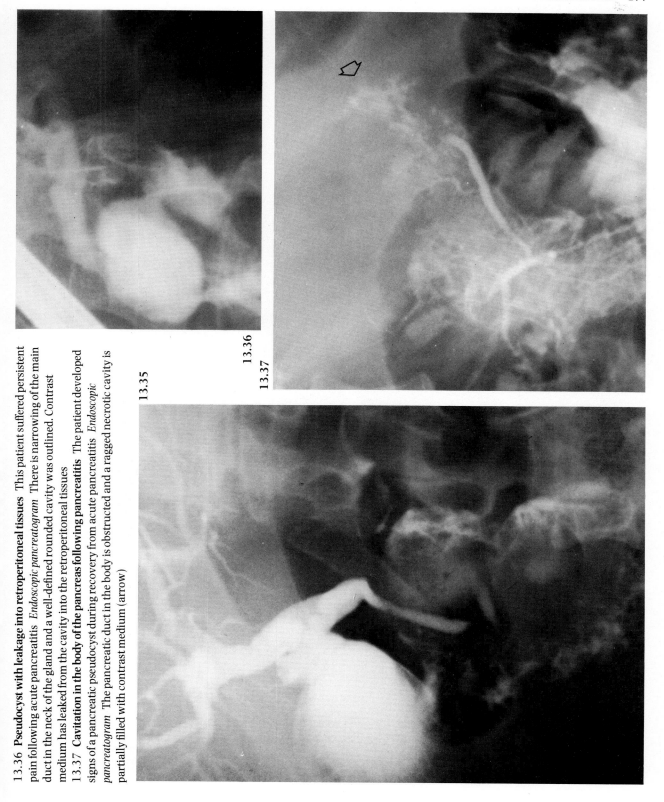

13.36 **Pseudocyst with leakage into retroperitoneal tissues** This patient suffered persistent pain following acute pancreatitis *Endoscopic pancreatogram* There is narrowing of the main duct in the neck of the gland and a well-defined rounded cavity was outlined. Contrast medium has leaked from the cavity into the retroperitoneal tissues

13.37 **Cavitation in the body of the pancreas following pancreatitis** The patient developed signs of a pancreatic pseudocyst during recovery from acute pancreatitis *Endoscopic pancreatogram* The pancreatic duct in the body is obstructed and a ragged necrotic cavity is partially filled with contrast medium (arrow)

13.35

13.36

13.37

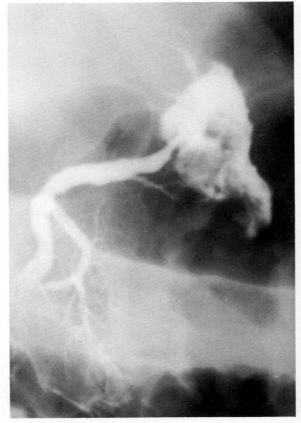

13.38

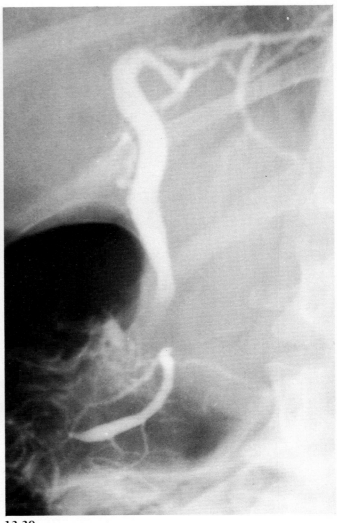

13.39

13.38 Pancreatic pseudocyst *Endoscopic pancreatogram* The main pancreatic duct is obstructed, and contrast medium has passed into an irregular cavity lying behind the stomach
13.39 Traumatic pseudocyst following blunt abdominal trauma *Endoscopic cholangiogram and pancreatogram* The main pancreatic duct is obstructed in the neck of the gland. At operation the pancreas was found to be ruptured and there was a large pancreatic pseudocyst which was not filled by contrast medium at pancreatography

13.40

13.40 Pancreatitis with unfilled pseudocyst compressing the common bile duct The patient was jaundiced *Endoscopic cholangiogram and pancreatogram* The pancreatic duct is obstructed in the neck of the gland. The lower common bile duct is compressed and there is dilatation of the intrahepatic and common hepatic ducts. The air-filled duodenum is indented by the swollen pancreas

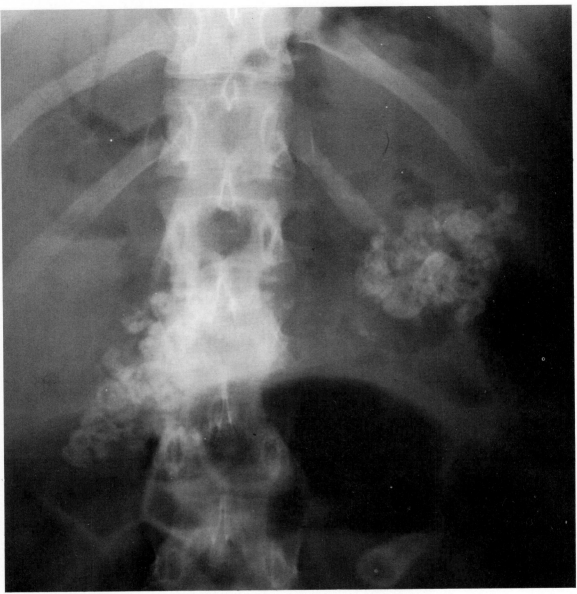

13.41

13.41 Pancreatic abscess in a patient with chronic pancreatitis *Plain abdomen (erect)* The film shows gas within an abscess cavity in the body of the pancreas, and concrements in the head and tail of the gland. Air is in the biliary tree due to a previous choledochoduodenostomy

Carcinoma of the pancreas accounts for about 5,000 deaths each year in the United Kingdom. There is evidence that the incidence of the disease is increasing, especially in men (Gordon *et al.* 1961). The disease most often affects patients in the sixth and seventh decades, and there is a male to female ratio in excess of 2:1. Chronic pancreatitis may be a predisposing condition (Bartholomew *et al.* 1958).

Two-thirds of pancreatic carcinomas have their origin in the head of the pancreas and histologically the great majority are adenocarcinomas. Except for the rare cystadenocarcinoma, pancreatic carcinomas are relatively avascular tumours which grow insidiously; symptoms do not usually develop until the lesion has exceeded the confines of the pancreas or involved the common bile duct. Obstructive jaundice, upper abdominal pain and loss of weight are the commonest symptoms, although some patients may present with late onset diabetes, pancreatic steatorrhoea or thrombophlebitis. Gastrointestinal bleeding of varying severity may occur.

Pancreatic carcinoma spreads readily to regional lymph nodes, especially by means of the peri-neural lymphatics, and may invade adjacent structures such as the duodenum, stomach, kidney and blood vessels. Liver metastasis is very common and pulmonary metastasis may simulate bronchiolar carcinoma or produce pulmonary lymphangitis carcinomatosum. Of considerable importance is the study of Mikal & Campbell (1950) which showed that of 100 necropsy cases 13 per cent. had no metastases and a further 5 per cent. had only local invasion; thus 18 per cent. were potentially curable. Successful excision of symptomless carcinomas confined to the pancreas found incidentally at laparotomy would suggest that the poor prognosis of carcinoma of the pancreas is due to delay in presentation and diagnosis. None the less the prognosis of carcinoma of the pancreas is extremely poor and the majority of patients are dead within a few months of diagnosis. Ampullary carcinoma and malignant insuloma have a somewhat better prognosis because they produce symptoms earlier in their course and before distal spread has occurred.

Cystadenoma is a slow-growing pancreatic tumour which occurs more commonly in women than in men and can reach a large size. Carcinoid tumours and sarcomata are very rare.

Insulin-producing beta-cell adenoma is the commonest cause of spontaneous hypoglycaemia. Ninety per cent. of insulin-producing tumours are benign; they are often solitary and may occur anywhere in the pancreas, although there is a relatively high incidence of occurrence in the tail. Gastrin-secreting non-beta-cell tumours may produce the Zollinger–Ellison syndrome (1955), about two-thirds of which are malignant and many have metastasized to the liver by the time they are diagnosed. Islet-cell tumours may be associated with adenomata in other endocrine organs (Zollinger & Grant 1964). Other benign tumours such as fibroma, lipoma and neuroma occur, but do not appear to be of any clinical significance.

The pancreas may become involved through malignant tumours which occur in adjacent organs such as the stomach and colon, or as a result of metastatic carcinoma.

Radiology

Plain radiography of the abdomen has little to offer in the diagnosis of

14 Tumours of the Pancreas

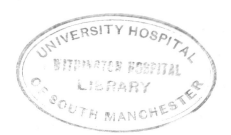

pancreatic carcinoma. Large masses displacing a gas-filled viscus or an enlarged gallbladder may occasionally be evident and the spleen may be enlarged if the splenic vein is occluded. Calcification is not a feature of pancreatic carcinoma, although disappearance or displacement of pancreatic calcifications by neoplasm have been observed (Tucker & Moore 1963). Calcification may be observed in the rare cystadenocarcinoma.

Barium examination   Barium studies may reveal suggestive abnormalities of the upper intestinal tract in 30 to 50 per cent. of patients (Smith *et al.* 1967; Moldon & Connelly 1968). With the exception of ampullary lesions, the tumours must be at least 3 cm in diameter to induce changes, and very much larger if they lie in the body or tail of the pancreas. The use of smooth muscle relaxants to promote visualization of the duodenal loop is increasing and has improved the diagnosis of lesions in the head of the pancreas. Intubation is not essential to produce good results and the hypotonic method can be included in the routine barium meal examination for patients with suspected pancreatic lesions (Kreel 1969).

The duodenal loop may be displaced, widened or deformed by a space-occupying lesion in the head of the pancreas. In addition, shallow filling defects and spiculated distortion of the mucosal pattern may be shown along the medial aspect of the descending duodenum. The epsilon sign refers to the barium outline of the medial aspect of the descending duodenum which is indented above and below the region of the papilla. This sign is seen when a large tumour invades the duodenum, but it may also be seen in pancreatitis. The presence of a filling defect with a cauliflower-like outline in the papillary region is more likely to indicate the presence of a neoplasm. Tethering, deformity and stricturing due to involvement by a tumour may also occur in the duodenal bulb or the third part of the duodenum, and the duodeno-jejunal flexure may be displaced downwards if the body of the pancreas is involved. Dilatation of the common bile duct above the neoplasm may produce a smooth indentation of the medial aspect of the descending duodenum above the papilla or an indentation across the apex of the duodenal bulb. Enlargement of the gallbladder may also cause a smooth lateral indentation on the duodenal cap.

The antrum is the most common part of the stomach to be involved by pancreatic tumour and may be displaced upwards or forwards. Mucosal abnormalities due to tethering and invasion may be evident on its posterior or inferior aspect. An increase in the width of the retrogastric space is a sign of a retrogastric mass which is difficult to evaluate because the space is so often widened in otherwise healthy obese or broad-bodied individuals. More indicative is the presence of a localized rounded impression on the posterior aspect of the body of the stomach. The stomach may be so extensively involved by an extrinsic pancreatic neoplasm as

to imitate intrinsic gastric carcinoma. Involvement of the cardia or lower oesophagus has been observed in patients with carcinoma of the body or tail of the pancreas.

Organ scanning   Selenomethionine pancreatic scanning and ultrasound scanning are two other non-invasive methods which are used to investigate pancreatic tumours. Assessment of the pancreatic scintiscan is difficult because the commonest finding in patients with pancreatic carcinoma is uniform impairment of uptake of selenomethionine. Localized impairment of uptake in the body or tail of the pancreas is seen in a minority of patients with carcinomas; similar impairment may be seen in pancreatitis and in 20 per cent. of subjects without pancreatic disease. None the less the examination can be useful because a subject with a normal scan is very unlikely to harbour a symptomatic pancreatic carcinoma (Agnew *et al.* 1976) and the concomitant liver scan may detect hepatic metastasis in a patient with a pancreatic tumour. In the main, the technical problems and the poor discriminatory value of this examination has been disappointing. Ultrasound is similarly beset with technical problems of overlying bowel gas or adjacent bone, although some workers claim an 80 per cent. accuracy rate in pancreatic carcinoma (Pietri *et al.* 1975). Computed whole-body tomography in the axial plane is now becoming available; it does not involve invasive procedures and may have much to offer in the diagnosis of pancreatic disease (Haaga *et al.* 1976; Kreel 1977).

Endoscopic retrograde cholangio-pancreatography   The recent development of fibre-optic duodenoscopy and retrograde pancreatography has improved the diagnosis of pancreatic carcinoma. In a series of 85 consecutive patients with suspected tumours, 37 patients with subsequently proved carcinoma were diagnosed correctly, 13 of whom had tumour at the papilla which was evident endoscopically (Baddeley & Salmon 1975). Pancreatograms in 19 patients revealed either tapered strictures or occlusions of the main pancreatic duct with dilatation of the duct above the obstruction when this was visualized. Contrast-filled pools within the tumour were evident in 3 patients. In 5 patients the pancreatic duct could not be filled, perhaps because of occlusion by tumour, but cholangiography revealed strictures of the common bile duct within the pancreas. In 4 of the 85 patients the investigation was not diagnostic because cannulation of the normal papilla was not achieved. A false positive diagnosis of carcinoma was made prospectively in 9 patients, 6 of whom were shown at laparotomy to have obstruction of the pancreatic duct because of chronic pancreatitis; a retrospective review of the films of these patients revealed minor changes of pancreatitis downstream from the occlusion or dilated side ducts adjacent to the occlusion. Occlusions due to carcinoma are most commonly tapered, but irregular, eccentric or abrupt occlusions may be observed. None of the patients with normal pancreatograms in the series has since been shown to have carcinoma. The overall accuracy rate of the series was 84 per cent.; the false positives (11 per cent.) occurred mainly in patients with pancreatic duct obstruction due to chronic pancreatitis and in 4 cases (5 per cent.) the examination was non-contributory. There was no significant complication due to the procedure. The value of pancreatic juice cytology is now under assessment.

Endoscopic cholangiography has reduced the need for percutaneous transhepatic cholangiography in patients with jaundice, but the bile duct may not always be visualized and in a small number of cases cannulation may be unsuccessful. In such patients transhepatic cholangiography using the fine needle technique may be performed.

Angiography   Pancreatic angiography is a procedure which can be performed relatively quickly and with minor discomfort to the patient. Occlusion, displacement and irregular stenoses of the pancreatic arteries are the commonest findings. A rich tumour circulation is unusual and suggests a diagnosis of cystadenocarcinoma. Islet cell tumours may produce a distinctive localized tumour blush which persists until late in the examination and angiography is diagnostic in 76 per cent. of patients (Madsen & Hansen 1970). Involvement of the splenic vein suggests malignancy. Initial reports suggested a prospective accuracy rate of from 30 to 70 per cent. for the diagnosis of pancreatic carcinoma (Nebesar & Pollard 1967), but the accuracy of the procedure has probably improved with the use of superselective catheterization of the branches of the coeliac axis. In view of the value of endoscopic methods, angiography is now best employed in confirming the diagnosis in doubtful cases and in determining the extent of the tumour, also involvement of major arteries and the splenic veins, so as to assess operability. Splenoportal venography may also be used to assess venous invasion by tumours.

Other investigations   Retroperitoneal, intraperitoneal and gastric gas insufflation combined with tomography in the axial plane have been used to outline pancreatic masses, but the procedure is very uncomfortable for the patient and the high index of suspicion required before the procedure is performed would justify diagnostic laparotomy. The diagnosis of pancreatic carcinoma might be considered a despondent exercise for in the above-mentioned series (Baddeley & Salmon 1975; Salmon 1975), only one of forty patients has survived for a year following apparently successful extirpation of a tumour which lay in the tail of the pancreas. However, retrograde pancreatography allows pre-operative diagnosis which may be of value, and it demonstrates the cause of symptoms in patients with other pathologies which simulate the disease clinically.

Some method of pre-symptomatic screening procedure would seem to be essential if the early diagnosis of pancreatic carcinoma is to be improved.

References

Agnew J. E., Maze M. & Mitchell C. J. (1976) *Brit. J. Radiol.*, **49**, 979

Baddeley H. & Salmon P. R. (1975) In *Abst. 3rd Cong. European Assoc. Radiol.*, p.150. Edinburgh: Churchill–Livingstone

Bartholomew L. G., Gross J. B. & Comfort M. W. (1958) *Gastroenterology*, **35**, 473

Gordon T., Crittenden M. & Haenzel W. (1961) *Nat. Cancer Inst. Monogr.*, **6**, 133

Haaga J. R., Alfidi R. J., Zelch M. G., Meany T. F., Boller M., Gonzalez L. & Jelden G. L. (1976) *Radiology*, **120**, 589

Kreel L. (1969) *Proc. roy. Soc. Med.*, **62**, 881

Kreel L. (1977) *Brit. J. Radiol.*, **50**, 2

Madsen B. & Hansen E. S. (1970) *Brit. J. Radiol.*, **43**, 185

Mikal S. & Campbell A. J. A. (1950) *Surgery*, **28**, 963

Moldon R. E. & Connelly R. R. (1968) *Gastroenterology*, **55**, 677

Nebesar R. A. & Pollard J. J. (1967) *Radiology*, **89**, 1017

Pietri H., Rosselo R., Serafino X. & Paoli J. (1975) *Proc. 8th Symp. European Pancreatic Club*, Toulouse

Salmon P. R. (1975) In *Eleventh Symposium on Advanced Medicine*, (Ed. Lant A. F.) p.55. London: Pitman Medical

Smith P. E., Krementz E. T., Reed R. J. & Bufkin W. J. (1967) *Surg. Gynec. Obstet.*, **124**, 1288

Tucker D. H. & Moore I. B. (1963) *New Engl. J. Med.*, **268**, 31

Zollinger R. M. & Ellison E. H. (1955) *Ann. Surg.*, **142**, 709

Zollinger R. M. & Grant G. N. (1964) *J. Amer. med. Ass.*, **190**, 181

14.1

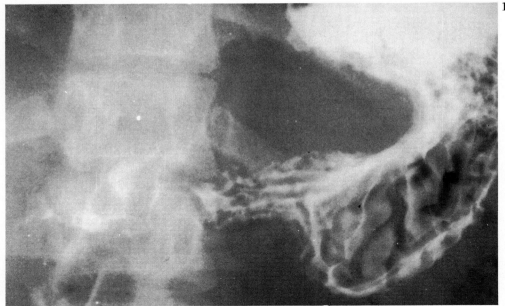

14.2

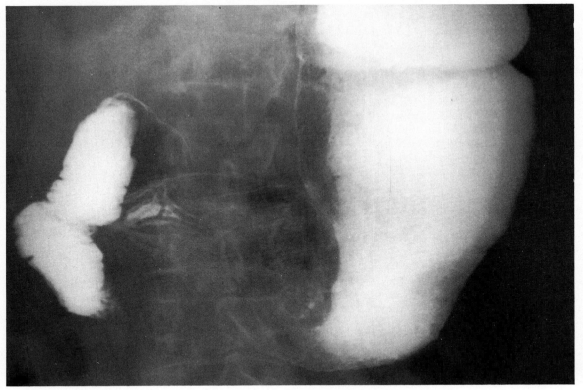

14.1 **Carcinoma of the head of the pancreas causing gastric outlet obstruction** *Barium meal* A large pancreatic carcinoma is indenting the greater curve aspect of the antrum of the stomach and invading the first part of the duodenum

14.2 **Carcinoma of the head of the pancreas causing duodenal obstruction** *Barium meal* The invading pancreatic carcinoma has grossly dilated the stomach, in which there is delayed emptying due to obstruction of the third part of the duodenum

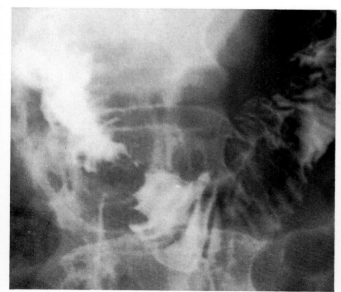

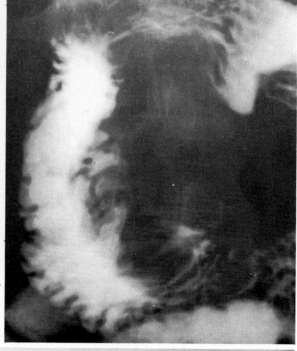

14.3

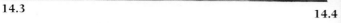

14.4

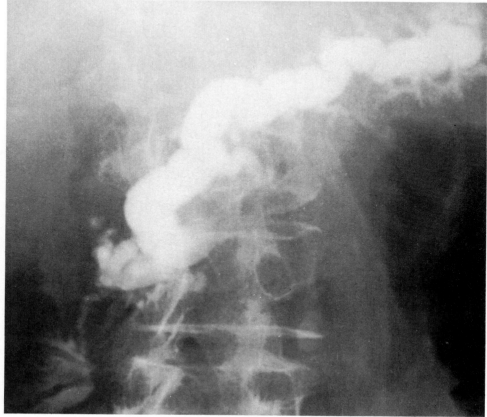

14.5

14.3 Carcinoma of the head of the pancreas invading the duodenum *Hypotonic duodenography* There is lobulated indentation of the medial aspect of the descending duodenum and a malignant stricture proximal to the inferior flexure due to invading pancreatic carcinoma.

14.4 Carcinoma of the head of the pancreas *Hypotonic duodenography* A large well-defined filling defect has arisen from the medial aspect of the duodenum due to carcinoma of the head of the pancreas

14.5 Carcinoma of the head of the pancreas *Endoscopic pancreatogram* A 3-cm-long irregular stricture of the main pancreatic duct occurs above the papilla. There is uniform dilatation of the main duct above the stricture

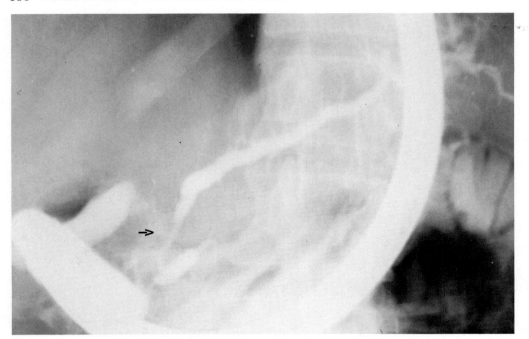

14.6

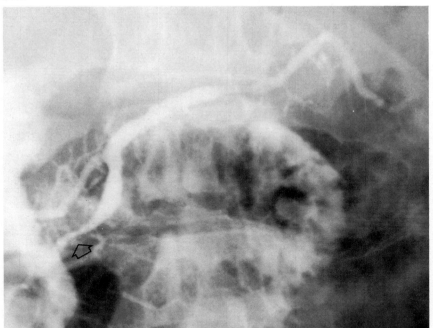

14.7

14.6 **Carcinoma of the head of the pancreas** *Endoscopic pancreatogram* There is a tapered stricture of the main pancreatic duct in the head of the pancreas with moderate dilatation of the duct above it

14.7 **Carcinoma of the head of the pancreas** *Endoscopic pancreatogram* A tapered narrowing of the main duct occurs in the head of the pancreas (arrow) due to encasement by tumour. The duct to the uncinate process is irregular and distorted. Gross dilatation of the main duct in the body and tail of the pancreas has been prevented by the presence of a patent Santorini duct

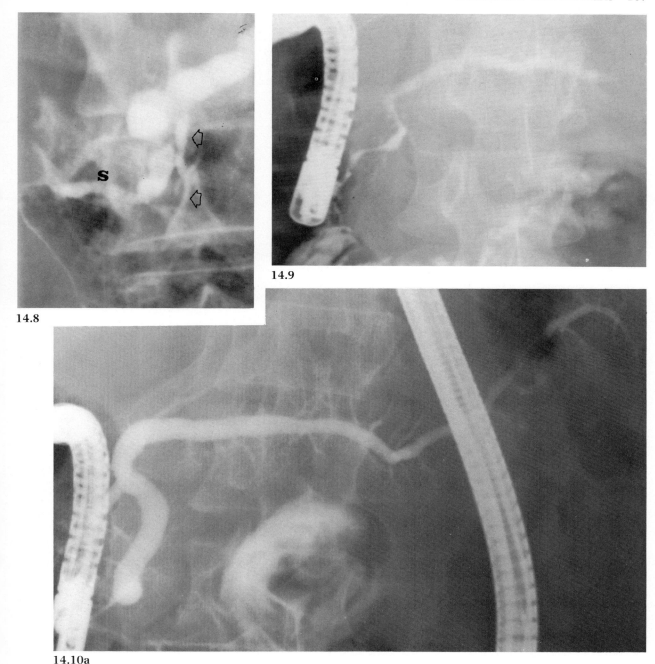

14.8

14.9

14.10a

14.8 Carcinoma of the head of the pancreas *Endoscopic pancreatogram* A stricture of the main pancreatic duct is caused by encasement with tumour (arrows). The main duct above the stricture and the Santorini ducts are dilated; the Santorini duct was blind and did not drain separately into the duodenum

14.9 Carcinoma of the head of the pancreas *Endoscopic pancreatogram* An irregular stricture of the main pancreatic duct is present in the head of the pancreas, with moderate dilatation of the duct in the body and tail of the gland

14.10 Carcinoma of the head of the pancreas a *Endoscopic pancreatogram* A tapered stricture of the main duct, 1·5 cm in length, occurs just proximal to the papilla, with moderate dilatation of the duct above the narrowed area. The biliary tree could not be filled. *(continued overleaf)*

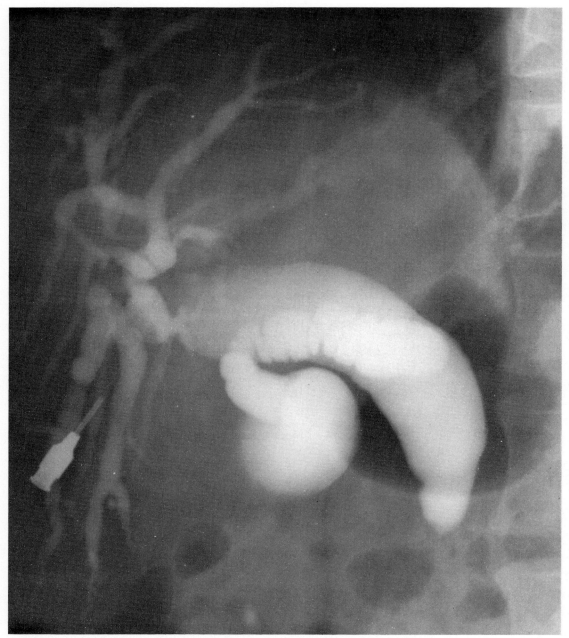

14.10b

14.10 b *Percutaneous transhepatic cholangiogram*   There is tapered obstruction of the lower common bile duct behind the pancreas and proximal dilatation of the biliary tree. A carcinoma arising in the uncinate process was discovered at operation

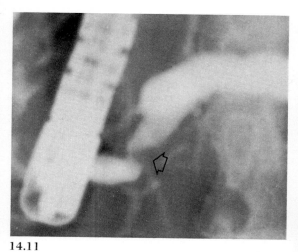

14.11

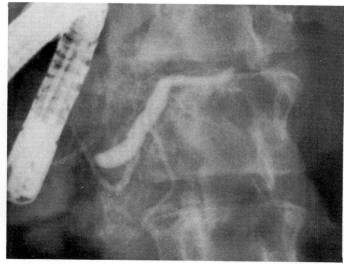

14.12

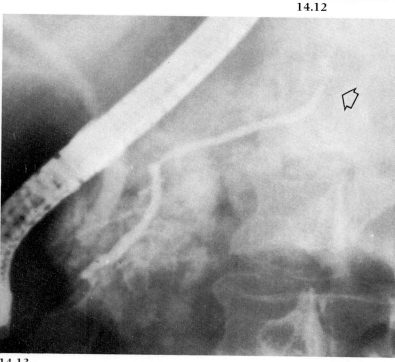

14.13

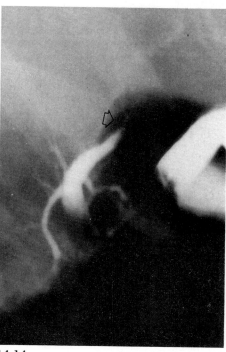

14.14

14.11 **Pancreatic carcinoma** *Endoscopic pancreatogram* A filling defect, 0·5 cm in diameter, occurs in the main pancreatic duct (arrow). At operation, the carcinoma was found to have spread beyond the confines of the pancreas, although radiologically the lesion appeared to be localized

14.12 **Carcinoma of the body of the pancreas** *Endoscopic pancreatogram* The main duct in the body of the gland is obstructed, but the ducts downstream of the obstruction are normal

14.13 **Carcinoma of the tail of the pancreas** *Endoscopic pancreatogram* The main duct in the body of the pancreas has a tapered obstruction (arrow). Some parenchymal filling has occurred downstream of the occlusion

14.14 **Carcinoma of the body of the pancreas** *Endoscopic pancreatogram* A long tapered occlusion of the main pancreatic duct has produced a 'rat tail' appearance (arrow)

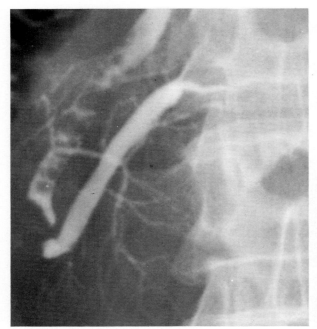

14.15

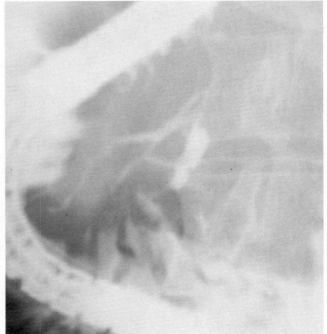

14.16

14.17

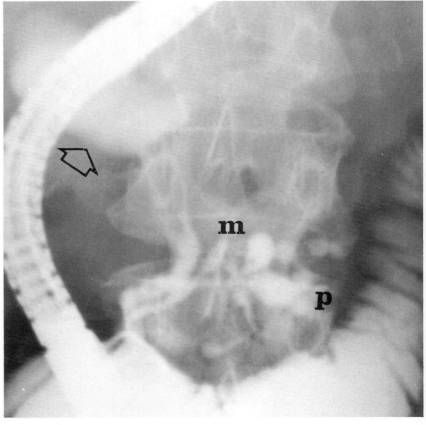

14.15 Carcinoma of the body of the pancreas *Endoscopic pancreatogram* A tapered occlusion of the main duct has produced a 'rat tail' appearance. The ducts downstream of the occlusion appear to be normal

14.16 Obstruction of the main pancreatic duct in the head of the pancreas by a carcinoma *Endoscopic pancreatogram* Although the main duct is occluded there is filling of ducts in the head of the pancreas

14.17 Pooling of contrast medium within a carcinoma of the head of the pancreas *Endoscopic cholangiogram and pancreatogram* The common bile duct (arrow) is dilated above a long stricture of the lower duct. The pancreatic duct is tapered and occluded 5 cm above the papilla *m*, and there are rounded pools of contrast medium within the carcinoma *p* (Salmon 1975)

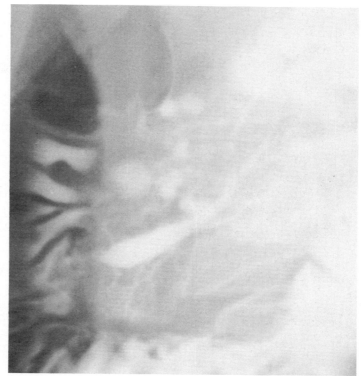

14.18

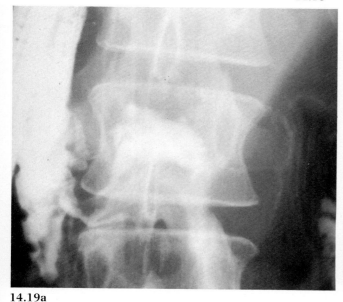

14.19a

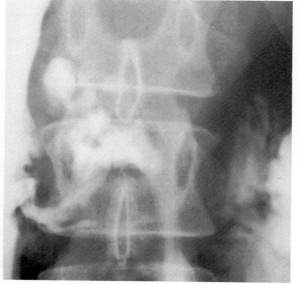

14.19b

14.18 **Pooling of contrast medium within a carcinoma of the head of the pancreas** *Endoscopic pancreatogram* The pools are round and interconnected and do not have the configuration or distribution of dilated ducts

14.19 **Cystadenocarcinoma of the pancreas** *Endoscopic pancreatogram* An irregular cavity in the head of the pancreas has filled, and the pancreatic duct has been replaced. Pools of contrast medium are present in the upper part of the head of the pancreas (Courtesy of Dr. J.F. Rey)

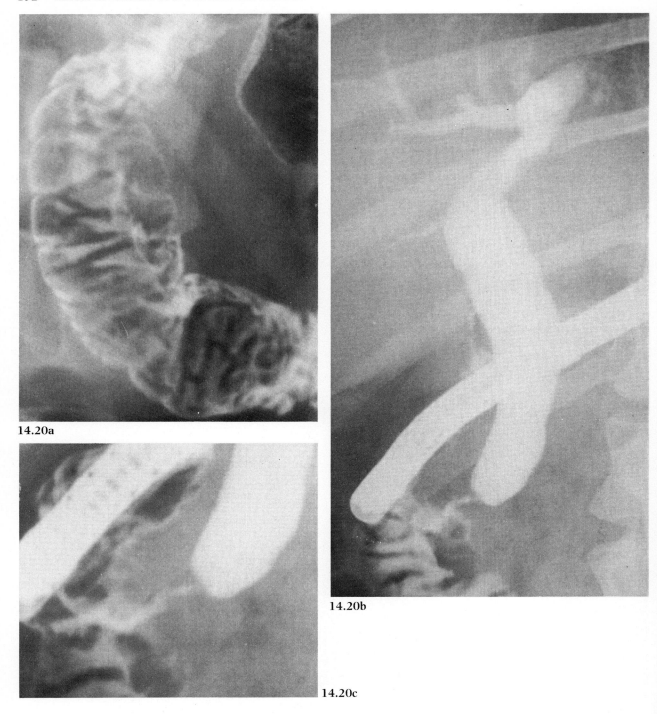

14.20a

14.20b

14.20c

14.20 Carcinoma in the head of the pancreas A 28-year-old man who presented with jaundice. a *Hypotonic duodenography* There is a filling defect of the medial aspect of the duodenum, even though the mucosa is intact radiologically and endoscopically. b & c *Endoscopic cholangiogram (no pancreatic duct filling obtained)* A 2-cm-long irregular stricture of the lower common bile duct is due to carcinoma. Failure of the pancreatic duct to fill was thought to be due to occlusion of the duct by a tumour

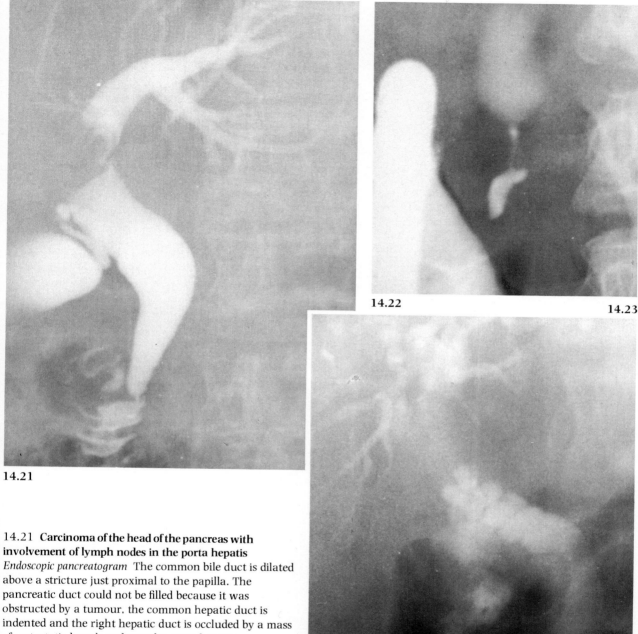

14.21

14.22

14.23

14.21 Carcinoma of the head of the pancreas with involvement of lymph nodes in the porta hepatis
Endoscopic pancreatogram The common bile duct is dilated above a stricture just proximal to the papilla. The pancreatic duct could not be filled because it was obstructed by a tumour, the common hepatic duct is indented and the right hepatic duct is occluded by a mass of metastatic lymph nodes at the porta hepatis

14.22 Carcinoma of the pancreas involving the lower common bile duct *Endoscopic pancreatogram* Occlusion of the pancreatic duct and a long irregular stricture of the lower common bile duct caused by carcinoma are shown

14.23 Carcinoma of the papilla *Retrograde cholangiogram* There is residual contrast medium within the dilated common bile duct following withdrawal of the endoscope. The lobulated upper border of the tumour has been well outlined

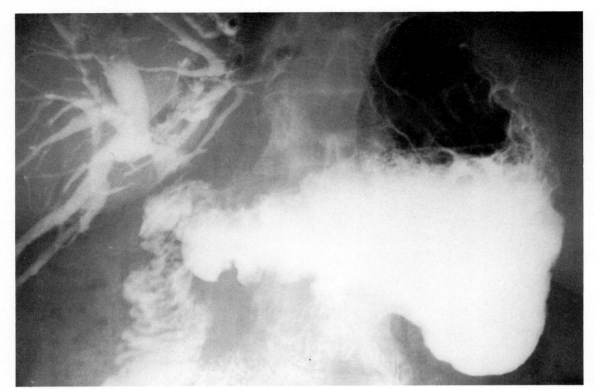

14.24a

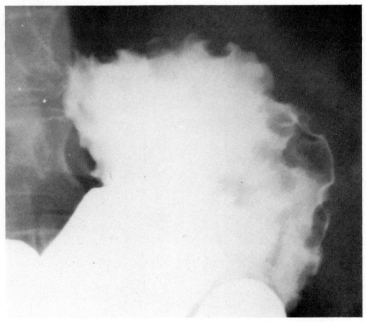

14.24b

14.24 Carcinoma of the pancreas involving the common bile duct and the splenic vein The patient presented with weight loss, anorexia and splenomegaly. a *Barium meal* The greater curve aspect of the antrum of the stomach is invaded by tumour and there is a choledochoduodenal fistula. b *Barium meal* Tortuous filling defects in the gastric fundus due to varices are demonstrated.

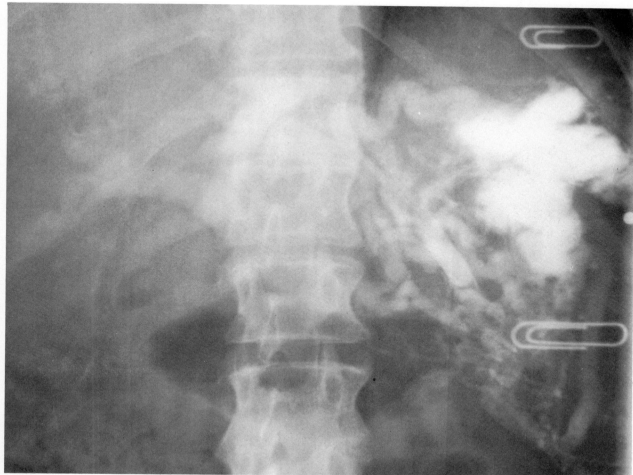

14.24c

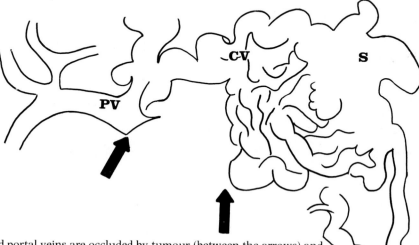

14.24 c *Splenoportogram* The splenic and portal veins are occluded by tumour (between the arrows) and a collateral venous circulation from splenic to gastric varices to the proximal portal vein is demonstrated. PV portal vein; CV collateral venous channels; S contrast medium injected in the spleen

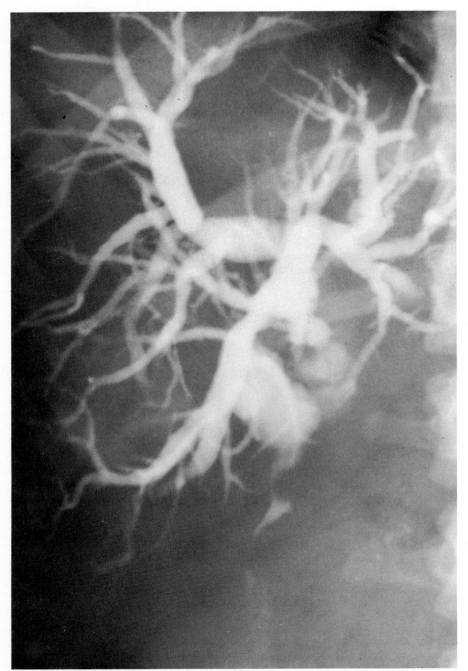

14.25

14.25 **Carcinoma of the pancreas occluding the common bile duct** The patient has had a cholecystectomy *Percutaneous cholangiogram* Lobulated filling defects are seen in the common bile duct, which is narrowed and occluded. The intrahepatic, common hepatic and remaining cystic ducts are dilated. No contrast medium has entered the duodenum

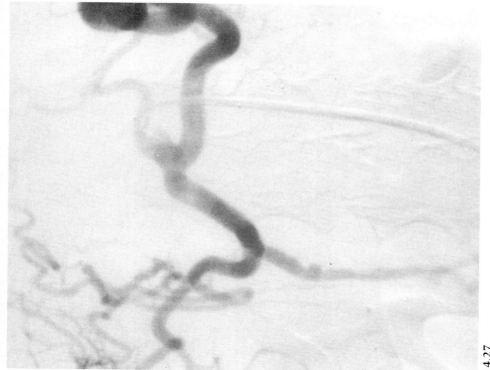

14.27

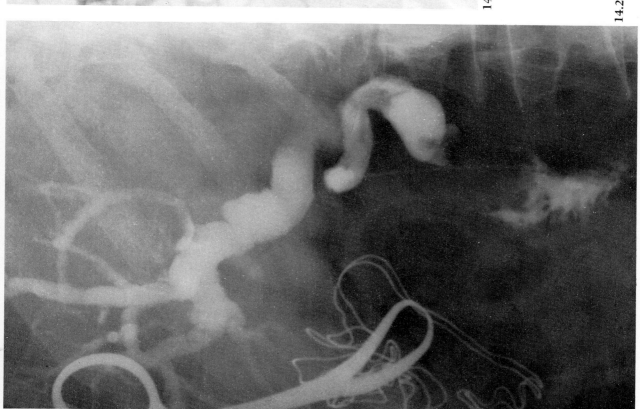

14.26 Carcinoma of the papilla *Operative cholangiogram* A large rounded filling defect at the lower end of the common bile duct protrudes into the duodenum

14.27 Carcinoma in the head of the pancreas *Coeliac axis arteriogram* The gastroduodenal artery shows irregular narrowing and encasement beyond its origin from the hepatic artery, caused by a carcinoma in the head of the pancreas (Courtesy of Dr. E.W.L. Fletcher)

14.26

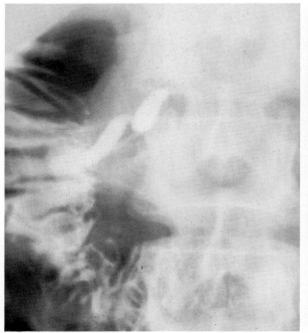 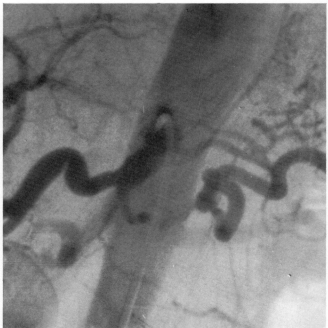

14.28a   14.28b

14.28 **Carcinoma of the body of the pancreas** This middle-aged patient complained of persistent epigastric pain and weight loss consistent with either carcinoma or pancreatitis. a *Endoscopic pancreatogram* The main pancreatic duct was dilated in the head and obstructed in the body of the pancreas, and there was poor filling of side branches. These appearances could have been due to neoplasm or inflammation. b *Coeliac axis arteriogram* There was encasement of the splenic artery and the branches of the dorsal pancreatic artery within the pancreas and a carcinoma was found in this position at laparotomy

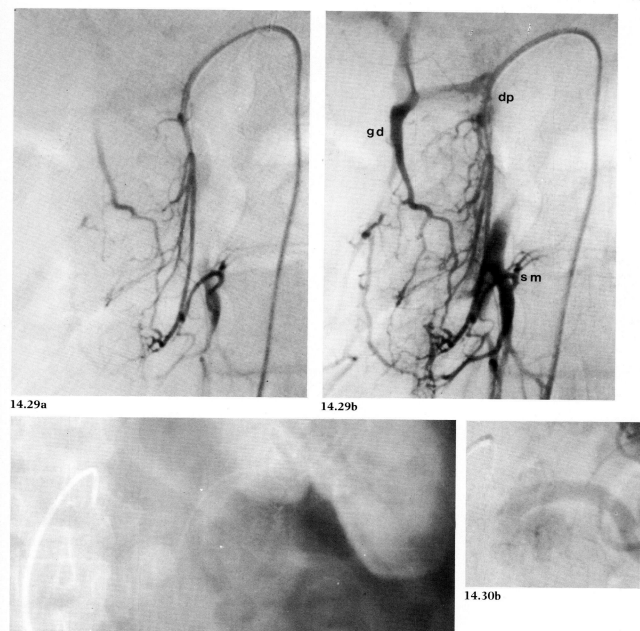

14.29a

14.29b

14.30a

14.30b

14.29 Carcinoma of the head of the pancreas *Superselective pancreatic arteriogram* a *Early film* b *Film later in the series* The catheter has been inserted into the dorsal pancreatic artery. The smaller arteries in the lower part of the head of the pancreas show irregular narrowing and encasement due to neoplasm yet the gastroduodenal *gd*, dorsal pancreatic *dp* and superior mesenteric *sm* vessels are not involved radiologically (Courtesy of Dr. H. Herlinger)

14.30 Insulin-producing islet cell adenoma *Coeliac axis arteriogram* a *Five seconds* The spleen is opacified and a well-defined tumour blush 1·5 cm in diameter is seen to the left of the L1–2 interspace. b *Subtraction of earlier film* The well-defined tumour lies just below the splenic artery in the body of the pancreas (Courtesy of Dr. E.W.L. Fletcher)

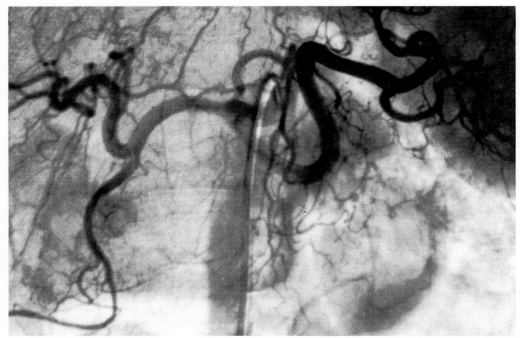

14.31a

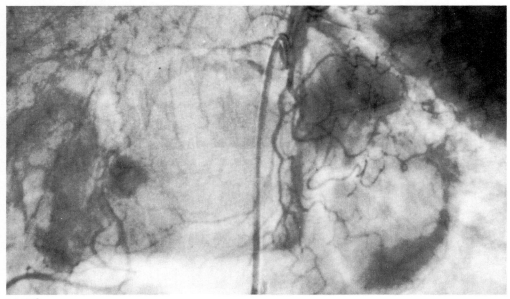

14.31b

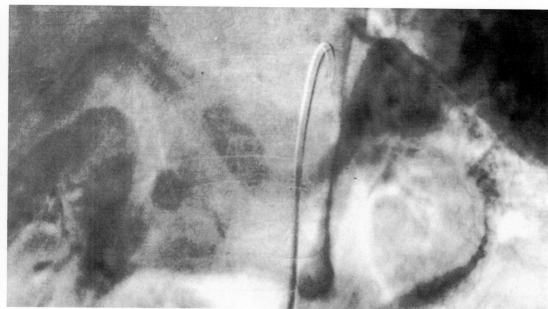

14.31c

14.31 Insulin-producing islet cell tumour The patient presented with fits due to spontaneous hypoglycaemia *Coeliac axis arteriogram* Subtraction films reveal a tumour blush in the head of the pancreas just medial to the gastroduodenal artery.
a *Arterial phase* b *Capillary phase* c *Venous phase* (Courtesy of Dr. E.R. Davies)

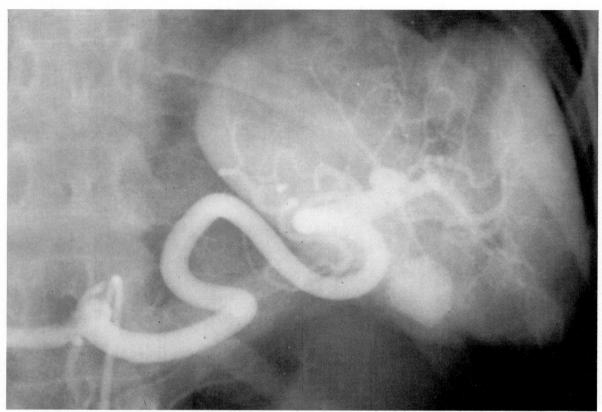

14.32

14.32 Insulin-producing islet cell tumour of the tail of the pancreas *Coeliac axis angiogram* The arterial phase shows a well-defined tumour blush adjacent to the spleen (Courtesy of Dr. E.W.L. Fletcher)

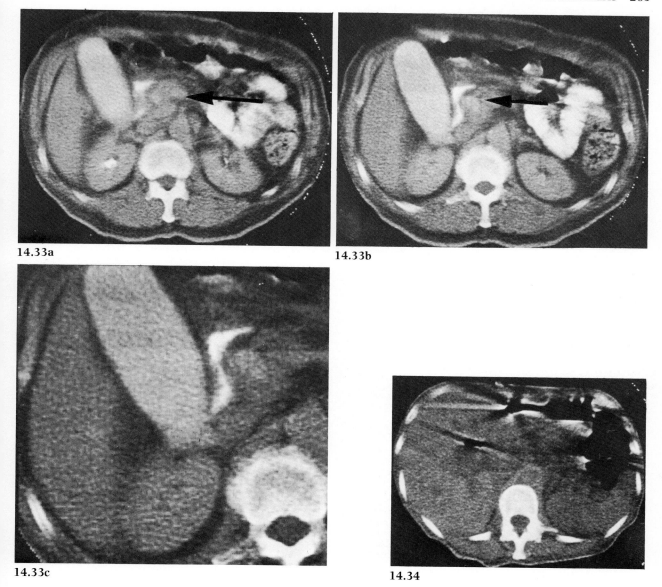

14.33 **Carcinoma of the head of the pancreas** *Computed tomography* a *Cut 7* The gallbladder is enlarged and opacified following recent cholangiography. Oral contrast medium outlines the small bowel in front of the left kidney and the duodenum which lies medial to the gallbladder. The mass in the head of the pancreas is due to carcinoma (arrow). b *Cut 6* The carcinomatous mass (arrow) is shown to indent the opacified duodenum on its medial aspect.   c *Magnified view of Cut 6*

14.34 **Carcinoma of the pancreas** *Computed tomography* A large carcinoma involving the head and body of the pancreas is outlined anteriorly by opaque contrast medium in the body and antrum of the stomach. The tumour has invaded and obliterated the peripancreatic and perivascular fat planes. The faint radiolucent areas in the liver are due to dilated intrahepatic bile ducts

Index